O YOU HAVE ROSTATE ANCER?

COMPACT GUIDE TO AGNOSIS AND HEALTH

D1636183

Dr. Emilia Ripoll, MD

Mark Saunders, MA

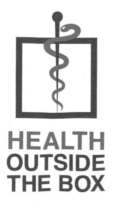

HEALTH OUTSIDE THE BOX

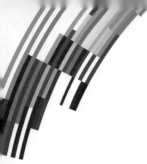

Emilia Ripoll, MD, Mark Saunders
Do You Have Prostate Cancer? A Compact Guide to Diagnosis and Health

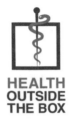

Vital Health Press/Health Outside the Box
6899 Countryside Lane, Unit 261
Niwot, Colorado USA
Health-OTB.com
info@health-otb.com

ISBN: 978-0-9962562-2-3
Library of Congress Control Number: 2016934818
Library of Congress Classification Number: RC280.P7
Dewey Decimal Classification Number: 616.99463

Subjects: Prostate-Cancer, Prostate-Cancer-Diagnosis

This 128-page book provides men who have had an abnormal prostate te?
digital rectal exam, or other lab test) with the most up-to-date information ?
prostate health, additional tests, and prostate biopsies. All the information
You Have Prostate Cancer? is presented in an easy-to-read format that m?
decision-making process simple and less stressful.

This publication is designed to provide accurate and authoritative informa?
regard to the subject matter covered. It is sold with the understanding that
publisher and authors are not hereby providing medical, psychological, fir?
legal, or other professional services. If expert medical assistance or couns?
needed, the services of a competent professional should be sought.

Cover Design by Just Designs
Inside layout & interior design by ZoeSnyder.com

Dr. Emilia Ripoll and Mark Saunders are available for speaking engageme?
quire about public speaking or bulk book purchasing email: mark@health-

Printed in the United States of America

TABLE OF CONTENTS

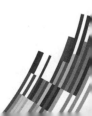

GRATITUDES & DEDICATIONS

Emilia's Gratitudes & Dedications

First and foremost, I dedicate this book to my husband, Tom, and my children, Marcos and Kiki, for putting up with me while working on this book.

I also want to thank my brother, Jesus, who taught me the value of my intellect and compassion, and gave me the opportunity to live, study, and work in the United States.

To Dr. Peter Scardino: Your brilliance as a surgeon and an academician coupled with your ability to connect with people on an emotional level set my standard for what it means to be a urologist.

To Dr. Dov Kadmon: I will always cherish your unwavering belief in me as a doctor and a healer. Thank you.

To Dr. James Jealous: You showed me what medicine was really about, reminded me of why I chose this healing path, and taught me innovative ways to care for my patients.

Last but not least, I would like to thank my co-author, **Mark Saunders,** and our graphic goddess, **Zoë Snyder.** I have been dreaming this book for years; you two allowed my dream to become a reality.

Mark's Gratitudes & Dedications

I dedicate this book to five men and three women:

To my father, Dr. Bartlett Saunders: In so many ways, without you, I wouldn't be here — neither would this book.

To Dr. Aaron Katz and Dr. Geo Espinosa: Without you two gentlemen, I might still be here, but my prostate would not. Thank you for launching me on this healing journey.

To John Fox and Ted Barrett-Paige: More than anyone will ever know, you two kept me sane as I went through my healing crisis.

To my co-author, Emilia Ripoll: I couldn't have done this without you, my sister from another mother. Bless you.

To Zoë Snyder: This book would be boring and drab without your incredible skill and persistence. Thank you.

To Sofie Trujillo-Shrock: Thank you for holding my hand and inspiring my heart. Your constant encouragement has made all the difference.

Zoë's Gratitudes and Dedications:

I wish to thank **Mark Saunders** and **Emilia Ripoll** for putting their faith in me to work with them on this project. Together we have created a valuable, and informative book that points people in a healthy direction.

We would all like to acknowledge **Anne Wood** for her early design contributions to this project.

Introduction
DO YOU HAVE PROSTATE CANCER?

" Everything should be made
as simple as possible,
but not simpler.

— *Albert Einstein*

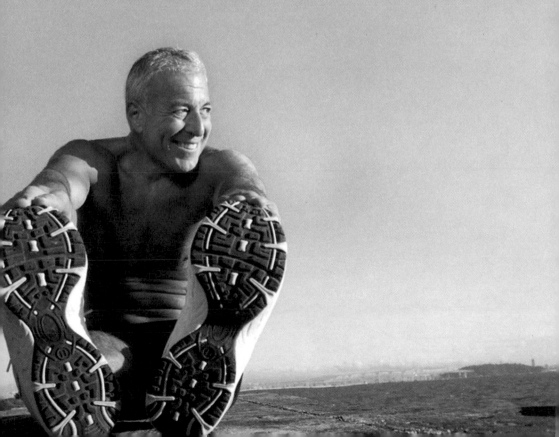

Patient Story

MARK

Prostates are tricky. They get a bad rap for being the little gland that brings big trouble. Maybe that's because we know so little about them.

As a 10-year prostate cancer survivor, I have come to see my prostate as a canary in a coal mine. I think of it as a barometer for my overall health & wellness, especially the health of all the organs in my pelvis.

If you are "sick in the prostate," then there's a good chance something's wrong with your overall health that prevents your immune system from kicking cancer's butt.

Here's a Top-5 list of what I've learned from prostate cancer in 10 years:

1. Listen to your intuition — especially when you don't like the message. That's the Big Kahuna talking.

2. Take an active role in your healing. Moving from cancer victim to cancer victor requires effort.

3. Take a 360° approach to finding the help you need. Be relentless. Explore unfamiliar territory. Never stop learning.

4. Doctors can work wonders, but you're the one who has to decide which treatment option is right for YOU. It's your body, your life, your decision!

5. Even though a prostate cancer diagnosis feels like getting whopped upside the head by the cosmic 2 x 4, if you are willing to embrace this healing challenge, it can be the gift that allows you to peel away the old patterns that no longer serve you and embrace the man you always wanted to be.

INTRODUCTION

If you're reading the introduction to this book (which many people skip), you're probably not lounging on the sofa on a quiet Sunday morning with cup of coffee, wondering if today would be a good day for a bike ride.

In order to be motivated enough to open this book, one of four events recently happened:

1. Your doctor told you that either a PSA test or a digital rectal exam (or both) found some areas of concern.

2. Someone you know was just diagnosed with prostate cancer.

3. Someone gave you this book because prostate cancer runs in your family.

4. You were diagnosed with prostate cancer.

Regardless of which of these events best describes your situation (or none of them), you're understandably concerned, perhaps even "freaked out." That's normal.

Since this book is about helping men gain a better understanding about prostate cancer and how it is diagnosed, let's skip the fluffy stuff and get down to it.

OUR GOAL

We seek to empower men to ask the right questions and make informed decisions. As advocates for prostate health and wellness, we do NOT have a stake in any diagnostic tests or treatments. Our only concern is that you choose the tests and treatments that are best for you.

OUR PURPOSE

We hope to provide men, their families, and their support network with the most up-to-date information about prostate health and cancer in an easy-to-read format.

This book is not intended as a stand-alone medical guide. Specific medical information about the health of your prostate should come from conversations with your healthcare providers. We encourage you to use this book as a point of departure for those discussions.

THE EVOLUTION A significant change in prostate cancer survival rates has occurred since the 1970s. Back then, 50 percent of the men who were diagnosed with prostate cancer already had metastatic disease (cancer that has spread outside the prostate, which is often fatal). Today, that number is less than 10 percent.

PSA blood testing is one of the primary reasons for this dramatic decrease in the number of men who have metastatic disease when they are first diagnosed.

PSA testing allows for early detection of the kind of prostate cancer that is likely to become metastatic disease. Since the early 1990s, PSA testing has saved untold lives and prevented needless suffering all over the world.

PSA testing remains a powerful tool in the battle against prostate cancer; however, it has its limitations. For example, elevated PSA numbers do not identify the culprit. Infection (prostatitis), enlarged prostate (BPH), and pelvic floor issues have raised the PSA of countless men who did NOT have prostate cancer, leading them to undergo unnecessary prostate biopsies.

Today, we are entering a new era in prostate cancer prevention, detection, and treatment. This next generation of prostate care provides doctors and patients with new tests and tools that pick up where PSA testing leaves off.

These tests and tools help doctors find hidden cancers and identify potentially deadly cancers while they are still in their infancy — when their cure rate is highest.

These new tests also identify men with low-risk, low volume cancers who do not need the same level of treatment as men with moderate-to-high risk cancers — effectively reducing the number of unwanted complications and side effects (See **Chapter 2**).

How This Book Is Laid Out

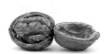

THIS BOOK IS DIVIDED INTO TWO SECTIONS:

THE BASICS | THE TOOLBOX

The Basics distills complex medical ideas and presents the information you need to know in a simple and direct way. This "in a nutshell" approach helps you understand the key concepts, ask the right questions, and select the best possible treatment for the kind of prostate condition you have.

The Toolbox is the interactive part of this book. It is a collection of tools that allows you to tailor the information presented in each chapter to fit your situation: assessment tools, checklists, worksheets, and questionnaires.

At the beginning of each chapter, you will find
- A Patient's Story of Surviving Prostate Cancer
- Chapter Summary
- Flow Chart
- Debunking Myths
- Vocabulary List

At the end of the each chapter, you will find
- A Doctor's Story about Prostate Cancer
- Looking Ahead
- What's Next
- **The Toolbox**
- "Notes" page

At the end of the book, you will find
- Glossary of terms
- Index

We encourage you to take advantage of these features. They can make the difference between choosing the right treatment option or making a decision you regret.

Regardless of whether you are reading a paper or electronic version of this book, it is **NOT** necessary to read this book "cover to cover."

Instead, we suggest you treat *Do You Have Prostate Cancer?* as a reference, like a mini-encyclopedia. Of course, there's nothing wrong with reading this book from beginning to end — it's just not required.

HOW TO USE THIS BOOK

We recommend you read as much or as little as you like about each topic, then go the **Toolbox** at the end of each chapter and plug in your information.

Each chapter is relatively short, full of diagrams and illustrations, and can be read in 20 minutes. This easy-to-digest format gives you the essential information you need — without overwhelming you with medical acronyms and words you cannot pronounce. Each **Toolbox** section takes between 5-15 minutes to complete.

After you read each chapter and complete the **Toolbox,** you will have a much better understanding of prostate health, prostate cancer, and what your next steps are.

For example, let's say you want to know more about PSA testing. Using the Index, you locate the pages on PSA testing. The **Chapter 2 Toolbox** allows you to record your PSA info plus results from other tests.

We also suggest that you write down your questions and concerns about PSA testing in the Notes Section at the end of **Chapter 2**. This way, you are more likely to remember your questions during your next medical appointment.

For more information about PSA testing, we recommend that you either purchase or ask your doctor for a copy of *Prostate Cancer: A New Approach to Diagnosis, Treatment, and Health.*

WE'VE DONE THE HEAVY LIFTING FOR YOU

If you Google "prostate cancer," you will receive about 30 million results. At 5 minutes per result, that's about 2.5 million hours of reading. You wouldn't have time to read them all, even if you lived to be 200 — and Google probably wouldn't be around by then anyway!

Instead of reading two dozen Google searches and feeling utterly lost, we have assembled the best-available information on the medical, surgical, psychological, and lifestyle aspects of a prostate cancer diagnosis — presented in a format that is free from scientific jargon and doctor speak.

As you read on, we will provide you with the ideal amount of information about the following topics:

- Innovative new tests and treatments
- The pros and cons of various testing options
- The different kinds of prostate cancer and how doctors distinguish one from the other.
- How to reverse the disease process going on in your prostate (and the rest of your body), and begin the journey back to health and wellness.

HEADS UP

Just by reading this introduction, you have embarked on a healing journey. Like all journeys, this one defies straight-line logic — one day you move ahead by leaps and bounds, only to slide backwards on the next. You'll also be thrown a couple of curve balls along the way. That's all part of this heroes' journey. And yes, restoring your health is heroic work.

REGAINING CONTROL

In order to heal from prostate disease (especially prostate cancer), you are going to have to make some major changes. Big changes are often accompanied by serious resistance — within yourself and from others. Why? Because change messes with the status quo and our sense of control. And most men like feeling in control.

The following is an example of how this book helps you to take advantage of leading-edge medicine and common sense prevention techniques to regain control of your life.

Clinically **insignificant** prostate cancer ("hidden cancer" that is usually only found in an autopsy) is a small cluster of slow-growing cells that are inactive and do **NOT** present an immediate health risk.

Around the world, men develop remarkably similar levels of clinically **insignificant** prostate cancer as they age — regardless of their race, ethnicity, economic status, genetics, lifestyle, career, country of origin ... and so on.

Most clinically **significant** prostate cancers (everything from low-risk to metastatic disease) are a red flag that some type of treatment is required: active surveillance, surgery, radiation, freezing the prostate, or some combination of treatments to destroy the disease.

Clinically **significant** prostate cancer rates vary greatly by race, ethnicity, economic status, genetics, country of origin, career, current country, vocation, diet, exercise, stress levels ... and a host of other factors.

WHAT DOES THIS DIFFERENCE TELL US?

The difference in the rates for these two types of prostate cancer speaks directly to the role that lifestyle and environmental factors play in developing **significant** prostate cancer — factors that you have a great deal of control over. For more information on this topic, see **Chapter 4**.

WHAT DOES THIS DIFFERENCE MEAN FOR A MAN FACING A PROSTATE CANCER DIAGNOSIS?

As **Figure Intro 1.1** on **Page 10** illustrates, the progression from healthy prostate cells to clinically **significant** prostate cancer is a two-way street.

The seven health factors we discuss in **Chapter 4** (diet, inactivity, stress, immune system, hormones, structure, and toxic substances) all have an impact on inflammation, which can make healthy prostate cells more likely to develop cancer.

Likewise, disease processes such as BPH (enlarged prostate) and prostatitis (inflammation) can also contribute to prostate cancer.

FACTORS WE ONCE THOUGHT OF AS "SET IN STONE"	FACTORS WE NOW KNOW TO BE "FLUID"
YOUR FAMILY HISTORY & GENETICS	• "Epigenetics" (gene modifications that do not involve genetic mutations) can change the expression of certain genes (small sections of DNA), and therefore the proteins these genes instruct the cell to make. These changes can affect both "tumor suppressor genes" (which protect against cancer) and "oncogenes" (which promote cancer). • 90% of prostate cancers are associated with "gene silencing" (a form of epigenetics that can shut down the genes that repair your DNA). Gene silencing makes it hard for cells to repair genetic modifications and mutations that contribute to cancer. • Folate, vitamin B12, tea polyphenols, genistein, and other foods can cause "epigenetic" modifications that turn these genes back on.
YOUR PAST	• Physical injuries to your lower back, pelvis, or legs can affect your prostate and pelvic floor and lead to prostate disease. • Many physical, emotional, and sexual traumas from your childhood and teenage years can turn certain genes on or off, which can lead to prostate disorders, including cancer. Healing physical and emotional trauma can change the expression of these genes (see above).
EXPOSURE TO ENVIRONMENTAL TOXINS	• Many of the chemicals that are known to promote prostate cancer (carcinogenic compounds) can be measured and treated with standard detox protocols and eliminated from your body. • You cannot control which chemicals you were exposed to before, but you can detox and limit your future environmental exposure.
BIOLOGICAL VS CHRONOLOGICAL AGE	• Diet, exercise and stress are the three biggest contributors to how young and vibrant your body looks, functions, and feels. A healthy diet, daily exercise, and a low stress levels all help prevent the initiation and promotion of cancer.
YOUR STRESS LEVEL	• Stress hormones are known contributors to the initiation and promotion of cancer. Identifying and changing stress patterns in your life can help you prevent the development of cancer and other diseases.
YOUR THOUGHTS	• Dwelling on recurring negative thoughts can increase your stress level; therefore, increasing the chance of developing all sorts of diseases, including cancer.

Figure Intro 1.0 lists a few "bedrock truths" that medical science once believed were fixed and permanent in individuals, which we now know are more plastic than previously thought.

7 FACTORS THAT DECREASE INFLAMMATION AND REDUCE THE RISK OF PROSTATE CANCER

1. Diet   2. Inactivity   3. Stress   4. Structure
5. Immune System   6. Hormones   7. Toxic Substances

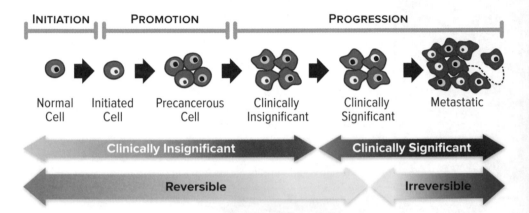

Inspired by Dr. Stephen Strum, Dr. Richard Beliveau and Dr. Denis Gingras, **Figure Intro 1.1** displays how plastic the process of developing prostate cancer is. Bottom line: Prostate cancer is treatable (and reversible) if caught early enough. Regardless of when prostate cancer is detected, one of the keys to reversing cancer's progress is eliminating the "hits" healthy prostate cells receive that spark the initiation, promotion, and progression of prostate cancer.

OUR CORE MESSAGE

The core message of this book is:
You can heal from prostate cancer.

The title of this book fits right in with our core message. The title asks, **Do You Have Prostate Cancer?** It is an important question for all American men, because one in seven men will be diagnosed with prostate cancer. This question is especially important for men who have received elevated numbers on certain tests.

If you are one of those men, just know that both of us have seen amazing recoveries from prostate cancer — true stories of healing from life-threatening disease.

For example, Mark has met two men who previously had triple-digit PSA numbers and now have PSAs of less than 1.0 with no signs of the cancer that once ravaged their bodies. (One of them had a four-digit PSA number.)

This type of healing from advanced prostate cancer is rare to be sure; however, the fact remains that your body is capable of incredible healing.

In fact, **your health never leaves you** — even if you have been diagnosed with prostate cancer.

One way to conceptualize this idea of your health always being there is to think about what happens to the darkness when you walk into a room and turn on a light. Once your health (the light) shines brightly, the darkness (disease) goes away.

If you turn your health light off again, the disease will likely return. That's not magical thinking; that's called "relapse."

We recognize that not every doctor you talk to will agree with us, and that's OK. It has been our experience, however, that men who are willing to embrace the challenge of changing their lifestyle and choosing the right type of treatment for their body and the kind of prostate disease they have (including cancer), a whole new world of possibilities opens up that they never knew existed.

With these thoughts in mind, let's begin the journey of healing your prostate and returning you to your rightful state of health and wellness.

Dr. Emilia A. Ripoll, M.D.
Mark Saunders, M.A.

Doctor Story

DR. SHANDRA WILSON, MD

Urology, Urologic Oncology
University of Colorado Hospital
Aurora, Colorado

As a surgeon, my favorite prostate cancer story is about a surgery patient, of course.

My patient is a lovely professor from Southern Colorado. He is a kind man who sports a thick ponytail and teaches students about college chemistry. My patient and his wife are one of those graceful couples who love people and express such gratitude for everything in their lives.

In 2006, this 50-something Ph.D. was diagnosed with aggressive prostate cancer and needed treatment. After extensive research (as one would expect), he decided to have a nerve-sparing prostatectomy at my hospital, which brought him to me.

The operation was difficult because of a previous pelvic surgery. I worked and worked to peel those delicate hair-like nerves away from his cancerous prostate.

When my patient came for his first follow-up appointment, he and his wife brought more than $300 of books for my children (who were 2 and 3 at the time). His wife, who is also a teacher, explained that the kindest thing anyone can do for a mom is to care for her kids.

She was right about that. My kids and I spent hours and hours reading and re-reading those delightful books.

Six months later, I received a Christmas card that said he had fully recovered and everything was working great. I sent him a card back.

Since then, we have developed a delightful friendship. My patient even says that he is "almost glad he got cancer," because it resulted in our friendship. I would never wish cancer on anyone, but I am in awe at how such a gift can come from something as horrible as cancer.

LOOKING AHEAD

CHAPTER 1: You or your doctor is concerned about your prostate — We provide you with **Prostate 101**: where it lives, what it does, plus relevant statistics.

CHAPTER 2: Your doctor told you to **schedule a prostate biopsy** — We give you a **Prostate Biopsy Assessment Tool** to see if you actually need one, and what to expect if you do.

CHAPTER 3: You have a prostate biopsy — We explain the steps you need to take, whether you have a **negative biopsy or a positive biopsy**.

CHAPTER 4: You want to **use your cancer diagnosis as a springboard to better health** — We help you address your wellness goals with a proven plan that covers inflammation, diet, inactivity, stress, immune system, hormones, structure, and removing toxic substances.

WHAT'S NEXT?

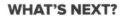

Where Do I Begin?
Go To Chapter 1

I Have NOT Had a Prostate Biopsy Yet
Go To Chapter 2

I Had a Prostate Biopsy
Go To Chapter 3

I Had a Positive (+) Biopsy
Get a Second Opinion

I Need More Information
Read
*Prostate Cancer:
A New Approach...*

WELCOME TO THE TOOLBOX
INTRODUCTORY **TOOLBOX**

In the Toolbox section at the end of each chapter, you will find question-naires, checklists, resource lists, assessment tools, and other interactive documents that are designed to help you put ideas into action.

The point of having a **Toolbox** section is to give you the opportunity to interact with the information presented in each chapter and make it personal and relevant for you and your situation.

Instead of one big Toolbox at the end of the book, we thought it would be easier to have a Toolbox section at the end of each chapter.

EACH TOOLBOX SECTION IS DESIGNED TO HELP YOU:

- Grasp what's going on inside your prostate
- Ask the right questions
- Make the most of your medical appointments
- Connect with your support team (or create one)
- Understand what your treatment options are
- Select the right doctor
- Pick the best possible treatment plan for you, your body, and the kind of cancer you have

---

The following Toolbox pages provide you with questions to ponder and space to write down your answers. The goal of the Toolbox section is to help you better understand your condition and give you a foundation of knowledge from which you make your medical decisions. We invite you to skip ahead and look at the other Toolbox sections to gain a sense of how this section works and what's to come.

TOOLBOX

7 FACTORS THAT DECREASE INFLAMMATION AND REDUCE THE RISK OF PROSTATE CANCER

1. Diet   2. Inactivity   3. Stress   4. Structure
5. Immune System   6. Hormones   7. Toxic Substances

PLEASE ANSWER THESE 8 QUESTIONS TO GET A REALISTIC VIEW OF YOUR HEALTH

1. How would you describe your diet? (Paleo, gluten-free, fast food ...)

2. What do you do for exercise?
(How often? How much time? How intense?)

3. How do you manage your stress?
(walking, singing in the car, meditation...)

4. Have you had any major physical injuries that required: surgery, physical therapy, osteopathic/chiropractic adjustments, acupuncture, or massage therapy? (circle one)   Yes   No   If "Yes," please describe.

5. Do you have an inflammatory medical condition like arthritis, diabetes, allergies, chronic infections, or other auto-immune disease? (circle one)   Yes   No

6. Are you taking (or have you taken) any medications that suppress your immune system? (circle one)   Yes   No

7. Have you been evaluated for low testosterone or any other hormone deficiency? (circle one)   Yes   No

8. Have you ever been exposed to toxic materials at home, school, work, or in your community? (circle one)   Yes   No

TOOLBOX

KNOW YOUR HISTORY

YOUR FAMILY HISTORY & GENETICS	Have any men in your immediate family (blood relatives) been diagnosed with prostate cancer? If so, at what age? Have any women in your immediate family been diagnosed with breast or cervical cancer? If so, at what age? Do you know if anyone in your immediate family has been diagnosed with the BRAC gene or other genetic markers?
YOUR PAST	Have you had any physical injuries that affected your lower back, pelvis, or lower extremities? (sports, car accident, fall on the ice) What kind of treatment, if any, have you had for these injuries? Do they still bother you today? Have you experienced intense emotional trauma? Loss of a child, parent, job, significant relationship, or other major trauma? (Circle one) Yes No
EXPOSURE TO ENVIRONMENTAL TOXINS	Have you been exposed to? (circle any that apply) • Radiation (medical or environmental) • Pesticides • Herbicides • Tobacco products or second-hand smoke • Hormones • Other toxic substances

TOOLBOX

KNOW MORE ABOUT YOURSELF

YOUR AGE (BIOLOGICAL VS CHRONOLOGICAL)	**YOUR CHRONOLOGICAL AGE AND BIOLOGICAL AGE MAY BE DIFFERENT.**
	
	1. How much energy do you have? (On a scale of 1-10, with 1 being little to none and 10 being abundant energy.)
	
	2. How flexible are you (physically and mentally)? (On a scale of 1-10, with 1 being very inflexible and 10 being very flexible)
	
	3. Do you exercise regularly (3 times/week or more)? (Circle one)
	    Yes No
	
	4. Does your body hurt most of the time? (Circle one)
	    Yes No
	
	5. Can you stand on one foot for 30 seconds without putting your other foot down? (Circle one)
	    Yes No
	
	6. How good is your memory? (On a scale of 1-10, with 1 being very poor and 10 being excellent.)

YOUR FUTURE	Are you excited to see what tomorrow brings? (Circle one)
	    Yes No
	
	Do you feel like your life is out of control? (Circle one)
	    Yes No
	
	Do you feel like your life has purpose? (Circle one)
	    Yes No

YOUR THOUGHTS	Do you spend more time thinking about what you want or what you don't want? What percentage of your time do you spend in worry or fear?

TOOLBOX

NOTES:

TOOLBOX

chapter ONE
Getting Started

What Cancer Cannot Do —
Cancer is so limited...
It cannot cripple love,
It cannot shatter hope,
It cannot corrode faith,
It cannot destroy peace,
It cannot kill friendship,
It cannot suppress memories,
It cannot silence courage,
It cannot invade the soul,
It cannot steal eternal life,
It cannot conquer the spirit.

— *Anonymous*

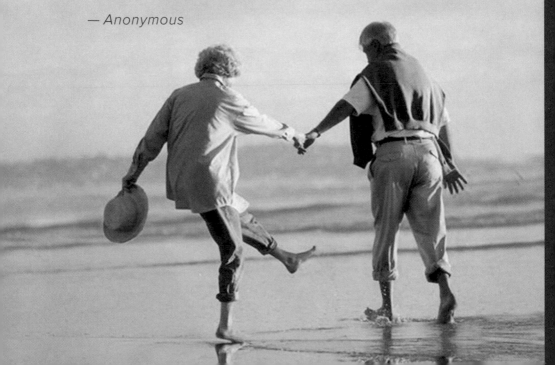

Patient Story

CLIFF

I was diagnosed with Stage 1 prostate cancer at the end of 2014, right before my 50th birthday. The first urologist I saw immediately recommended a radical prostatectomy, and also mentioned that radiation treatment was another option. I initially thought, "Sure. I don't need this organ to live."

Then I found out about the possible side effects of the surgery, including being impotent and incontinent — for the rest of my life!

I did some research, and what I learned gave me permission to try other options.

I eliminated sugars (including alcohol), dairy, meat, gluten and soy from my diet (and added apricot seeds, cannabis oil, apple cider vinegar and blackstrap molasses), and my weight dropped from 208 to 185 in two months (23 pounds). I started addressing my stress level, going to a holistic doctor, using a far-infrared heating pad, getting monthly acupuncture treatments, and taking dried Chinese herbs and mushrooms daily.

My PSA dropped dramatically, but I still had this one big nagging issue: How could I be sure the cancer wasn't growing?

From my research, I didn't believe I needed an annual prostate biopsy, as they can have negative side-effects too.

I am now working with a urologist who supports my choices, and I feel great! I have a goal of living to 90, and I want to celebrate the second half of my life by being healthy. If I eventually need surgery or radiation, that's fine — but I have made it a priority to not let my health get to that point.

chapter
ONE
summary

Chapter 1 introduces you to your prostate: where it is located, what it does, as well as some important information about prostate cancer.

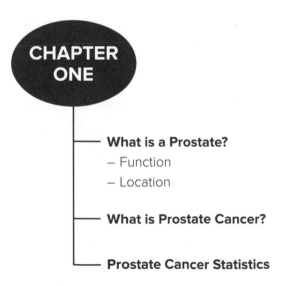

Figure 1.0 Illustrates the three major topics covered in Chapter 1.

DEBUNKING MYTHS

NO TWO CANCERS ARE IDENTICAL

Just as no two people are biologically the same, no two men have exactly the same kind of prostate cancer, which explains why one type of treatment may work perfectly for one man and poorly for another.

That's why it's so important to select a doctor who is an expert in prostate cancer and understands the pros and cons of pairing an individual who has a specific kind of prostate cancer with a particular type of treatment. This approach is the opposite of a doctor who performs the same procedure regardless of the patient or what kind of cancer he has.

The purpose of this book is to help you find the right treatment for the type of prostate problem you have (including cancer). Ideally, this treatment is powerful enough to eliminate the problem while preserving normal bowel, bladder, urinary, and erectile function.

Also, we do NOT have a stake in any procedures, products, tests, or medications. We just want you to be well.

VOCABULARY

See Glossary for Definitions

Bladder

Bio-individuality

BPH
(Benign Prostatic Hyperplasia)

Digital Rectum Exam (DRE)

DNA (deoxyribonucleic acid)

Gene

Gleason score

Hormones

Mutation

Pelvic Floor

Prostate Biopsy

Prostate Cancer

Prostate Zones

PSA (Prostate Specific Antigen)

PSA Testing

Rectum

Seminal Vesicle Fluid

Seminal Vesicles

Urethra

Urinary Retention

Urinary Sphincter

Urinary Stricture

THE LAY OF THE LOINS

Before discussing whether a prostate biopsy is right for you (**Chapter 2**), we would like to give you a short course in prostate anatomy and physiology, clarify a few terms, and provide you with the information you need to know to become an informed patient.

WHERE IS YOUR PROSTATE GLAND LOCATED?

Found only in men, the prostate is a walnut-shaped gland located below the bladder, behind the muscular wall of the abdomen, in front of the rectum at the bottom of the pelvis (See **Figure 1.1**). Since the prostate rests up against the rectum, the easiest way to access the prostate is by a digital rectal exam (DRE — See **Page 45**).

The tube that allows urine to drain from the bladder and out the penis (the urethra) passes through the middle of the prostate. One way to think of the prostate gland is that it's like a spongy golf ball with a straw running through the middle of it.

Your prostate surrounds your urethra and sits in between your bladder and urinary sphincter (See **Figure 1.1**). If there's congestion or blockage in the prostate (an enlarged prostate, a prostate cancer tumor) or below it (tight urinary sphincter or scar tissue in the urethra) urine can back up, causing varying degrees of pain and urine retention.

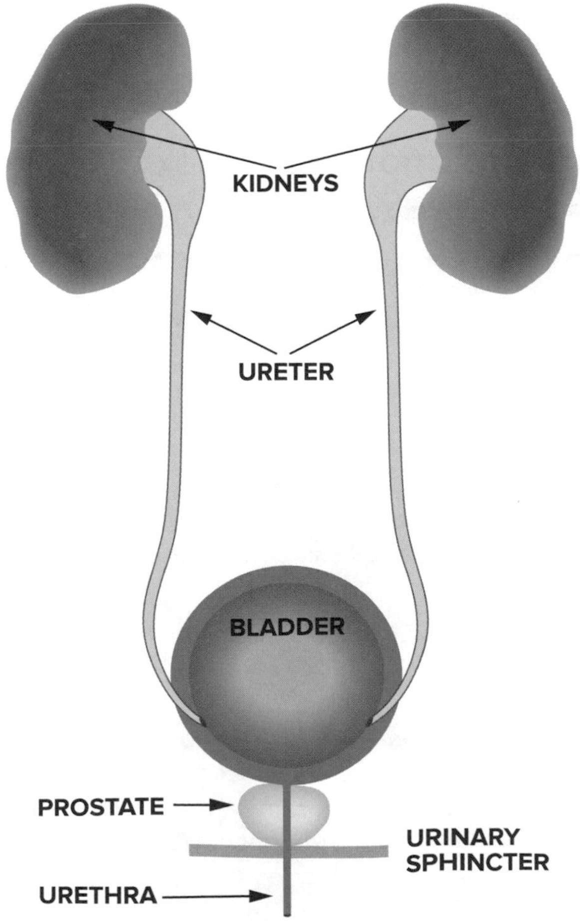

KIDNEYS

URETER

BLADDER

PROSTATE

URINARY SPHINCTER

URETHRA

Figure 1.1 shows the prostate gland in relationship to the rest of the urinary system.

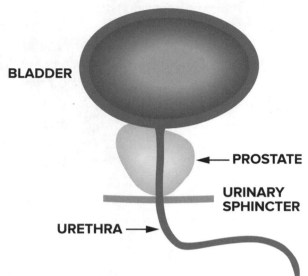

BLADDER

PROSTATE

URINARY SPHINCTER

URETHRA

Figure 1.2 shows a slice of the lower urinary system, with the bladder on top of the prostate and the muscular hammock of the pelvic floor/urinary sphincter below. An enlarged prostate, urinary strictures (scar tissue inside the urethra), or a tight urinary sphincter can cause urine to back up into the prostate, which may lead to inflammation and symptoms that mimic prostate cancer.

URINARY RESTRICTION AND BLOCKAGE

There are four main causes of urinary restriction and blockage:

1. *Enlarged prostate (BPH)*
2. *Tight urinary sphincter (pelvic floor dysfunction)*
3. *Urethral strictures (scar tissue in the urethra)*
4. *Prostate cancer*

Both an enlarged prostate and prostate cancer can cause urinary restriction and blockage within the prostate. A tight pelvic floor/urinary sphincter pinches the urethra just below the prostate. Urethral strictures can occur anywhere along the urethra.

Regardless of what causes the blockage/restriction, if it occurs "downstream" from the prostate, urine will back up into the glands of the prostate.

Since the urine of most Americans has a pH of 5 (the same acidity as black coffee), a urinary restriction or blockage is like soaking your prostate and urethra in a cup of black coffee all day and night. No wonder men with urinary restriction/blockage feel a painful, itching, burning sensation in their prostates.

WHAT DOES YOUR PROSTATE GLAND DO?

THE PROSTATE HAS TWO MAIN FUNCTIONS:

1. It secretes and stores the fluid that contains Prostate Specific Antigen (PSA), which acts like the "semen solvent" that allows individual sperm to swim on their own, instead of sperm clumping together in groups and spinning in circles.

2. The smooth muscles of the prostate contract during ejaculation, propelling semen down the urethra and out of the body during orgasm.

Like all the glands and organs in the pelvis, the prostate is affected by the health of the supporting structures, particularly the abdominal muscles, the lumbosacral spine, and the hammock of muscles and connective tissue that forms the pelvic floor/urinary sphincter.

ZONES OF THE PROSTATE

The prostate is composed of three main zones: Central, Transitional, and Peripheral. (See **Figure 1.3**)

The Central Zone surrounds the ejaculatory ducts and accounts for approximately 25 percent of the prostate volume. Only 2.5 percent of prostate cancers occur in the Central Zone; however, these cancers are usually more aggressive and invade the seminal vesicles.

The Transitional Zone, which surrounds the urethra in the middle of the gland, accounts for only 5 percent of total prostate volume at puberty; however, this portion of the prostate continues to grow throughout a man's life and is responsible for an enlarged prostate (BPH). Approximately, 10-20 percent of prostate cancer occurs in this zone.

The Peripheral Zone contains most of the "glandular" tissue in the lower half of the prostate, and surrounds the urethra as it leaves the prostate. This zone accounts for a whopping 70-80 percent of prostate cancer and is the most easily accessible by a DRE.

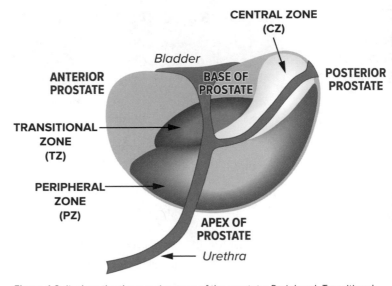

Figure 1.3 displays the three main zones of the prostate: Peripheral, Transitional, and Central.

WHAT CAUSES PROSTATE CANCER?

It is difficult to isolate a single cause of prostate cancer. We know that certain inherited DNA mutations (BRCA1, BRCA2, RNASEL, MLH1, MSH2) as well as mutations that occur during a man's lifetime can cause prostate cancer. Inherited DNA mutations appear to cause only 5-10 percent of prostate cancers. This means that mutations that occur after birth account for the other 90-95 percent of the prostate cancer cases.

If you look at **Figure Intro 1.1** on **Page 10**, you'll see that it takes multiple "hits" to prostate cells before cancer can find a foothold. It is important to realize that these hits come from the aspects of our lives that we can control (diet, exercise, stress management) as well as those we cannot (your family history & exposure to toxic chemicals).

WHAT DOES THAT TELL US?

If you're a pessimist, **Figure Intro 1.1** is proof that life is out to get you. If you're an optimist, it is proof that you have a lot more control over your health in general, and your prostate health in particular, than you thought possible.

In **Chapter 4,** you will learn more about how your diet, activity level, stress, immune system, hormone levels, structure, and exposure to toxic substances impact your overall health — and the health of your prostate.

WHAT IS PROSTATE CANCER?

Cancer happens when cells begin to grow in an out-of-control way. Normal cells grow, divide, and die in a predictable manner. Cancer cells, on the other hand, lose the ability to self-regulate, stop communicating with other cells, replicate faster than normal cells, and simply refuse to die. In fact, under the right laboratory conditions, cancer cells can live in Petri dishes for decades.

This hard-to-kill quality is what allows prostate cancer to invade territory beyond the prostate gland — lymph nodes, seminal vesicles, bladder, rectum, nearby bones, and eventually the entire body.

For more information on the risk factors for prostate cancer cells, see **Chapter 2.**

It is generally accepted that cancer is caused by a change (mutation or modification) of a cell's DNA (genetic code) that occurs while the cell is dividing and replicating. Once a mutation/modification occurs (assuming it doesn't kill the cell), it is passed on to all future copies of that cell.

Prostate Cancer can be seen as the result of microscopic changes to a small section of a cell's genetic code (genes) that increase the rate at which cells divide and replicate. Theoretically, turning these genes off — or turning on other genes that slow down the rate of cell division and replication — could stop prostate cancer from spreading.

Mutations/modifications can also control a cell's ability to repair itself. "Gene silencing" prevents a cell's microscopic mechanics from repairing the cell's DNA. When this happens, a cell can be overrun by invading molecules from nearby cancer cells.

Obviously, a lot of research is going on in these areas.

NOTE

In the United States, 15 percent of men will be diagnosed with prostate cancer during their lifetime. That information says nothing about which 1-in-7 men will develop prostate cancer. More importantly, it ignores who the other six are and why they were spared from this disease (or at least the diagnosis).

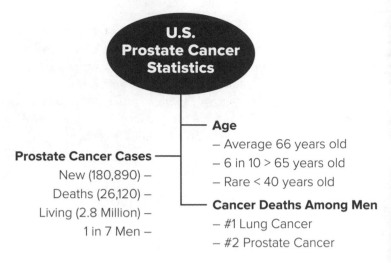

Figure 1.4 outlines the American Cancer Society's 2016 prostate cancer statistics. Notice that the 2016 numbers are all lower than the 2015 numbers.

PROSTATE CANCER STATISTICS

Here are the American Cancer Society's prostate cancer estimates for 2016. (All of these numbers are better than the 2015 numbers):

- New cases of prostate cancer (all ages): 180,890 (down from 220,800 in 2015). Approximately 1 in 7 men in the United States will be diagnosed during his lifetime.
- Prostate cancer has the highest incidence rate of all cancers in the United States: 131.5/100,000 men.
- Death from prostate cancer (all ages): 26,120 (down from 27,545 in 2015). Between 2008-2012, approximately 21 out of 100,000 men in living in the United States died of prostate cancer.
- Prostate cancer is the second leading cause of cancer death in American men; lung cancer is number 1. About 1 man in 38 will die of prostate cancer (2.6%).
- Prostate cancer occurs mainly in older men. About 6 out of 10 cases are diagnosed in men aged 65 or older, and it is rare before age 40. The average age at the time of diagnosis is 66.
- Race is a factor: African American men are more than twice as likely to develop prostate cancer than white American men — and more than twice as likely to die from prostate cancer.
- The probability of a man developing prostate cancer (and dying from prostate cancer) increases with age.

- Between 2005-2011, the 5-year prostate cancer survival rate for all-stages was 99%. The rate was more than 99% for cancer still inside the prostate; however, for cancer that had spread throughout the body (metastatic disease), the 5-year survival rated dropped to 28%.

Thanks to PSA testing, early detection, and better care, fewer men are dying of prostate cancer. For example, between 2008-2012, 21.4 out of 100,000 U.S. men died from prostate cancer, compared to 39.2 per 100,000 men in 1992, just before PSA testing became widespread. That's a **83 percent improvement!**

In addition to the statistics about new prostate cancer cases and deaths, statistics are available for each risk factor, type of prostate cancer treatment, and the complications of those treatments.

BIO-INDIVIDUALITY AND PROSTATE CANCER

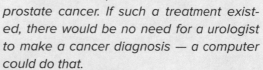

The term bio-individuality means that no two people are biologically the same (even identical twins). So it shouldn't come as a surprise that there is no one-pill-cures-all treatment for

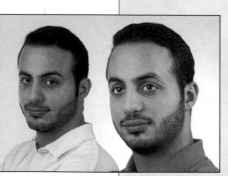

prostate cancer. If such a treatment existed, there would be no need for a urologist to make a cancer diagnosis — a computer could do that.

Bio-individuality isn't just an interesting idea; it is leading-edge cancer research. Dr. Steven Rosenberg, M.D. and his colleagues at the National Cancer Institute have developed a new form of immunotherapy (a way of enhancing the body's immune system) that targets the specific mutations (changes in a cell's DNA) of a particular person's cancer.

This form of cancer therapy (which is currently in Phase 1 and Phase 2 trials) creates a completely individualized form of treatment that kills 100 percent of the cancer cells and leaves all the other cells (cells that lack a cancer-specific mutation) alone. Dr. Rosenberg's therapy goes right to the heart of the question behind all prostate cancer research: How can we destroy all the cancer while sparing the healthy tissue around it?

The answer to that question is what keeps urologists up at night.

Doctor Story
DR. ELIZABETH CEILLEY, MD

Radiation Oncology

Banner Health

Loveland, Colorado

No matter how sophisticated the technology, or how precise the treatment plan, patients' experiences are shaped predominately by their interactions with their medical team.

My colleagues like to tease radiation oncologists like me about our love of "fancy toys." As my colleagues would expect, I was thrilled that our center was among the first to acquire a new TrueBeam STx Linear Accelerator. Our center was already known for its warm environment and caring staff. Now we were going to be a state-or-the art radiation oncology center.

The first patient to be treated by this new machine was "AA," a gentleman who had previously had a prostatectomy. His PSA was now rising and radiation therapy was recommended. Our hospital wanted to publicize our new technology, and AA was the perfect first patient because the technical aspect of his treatment was greatly improved by the True Beam Linear Accelerator.

However, AA was less than excited about being the first patient on the new machine. "I don't buy new cars for a reason," he said. He was also bothered by all the attention surrounding his treatment. Eventually, I recommended that a local magazine interview another patient for an article about our new linear accelerator.

AA's seven weeks of radiation treatment went well. In follow-up, he was doing great, and his PSA was undetectable. I later suggested that someone on our PR staff might want to interview AA about his experience.

When AA was asked for an interview, he said "Yes," and then added, "It was not that machine that made my treatment successful — it was the PEOPLE."

LOOKING AHEAD

CHAPTER 1: You or your doctor is concerned about your prostate — We provide you with **Prostate 101**: where it lives, what it does, plus relevant statistics.

CHAPTER 2: Your doctor told you to **schedule a prostate biopsy** — We give you a **Prostate Biopsy Assessment Tool** to see if you actually need one, and what to expect if you do.

CHAPTER 3: You have a prostate biopsy — We explain the steps you need to take, whether you have a **negative biopsy or a positive biopsy**.

CHAPTER 4: You want to **use your cancer diagnosis as a springboard to better health** — We help you address your wellness goals with a proven plan that covers inflammation, diet, inactivity, stress, immune system, hormones, structure, and removing toxic substances.

WHAT'S NEXT?

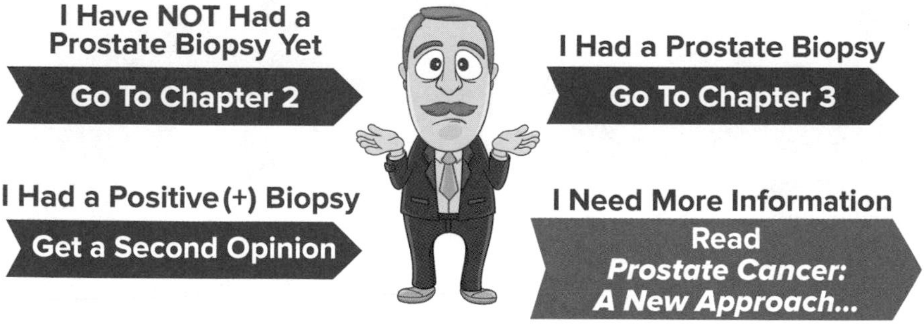

I Have NOT Had a Prostate Biopsy Yet
Go To Chapter 2

I Had a Prostate Biopsy
Go To Chapter 3

I Had a Positive(+) Biopsy
Get a Second Opinion

I Need More Information
Read
*Prostate Cancer:
A New Approach...*

WELCOME TO THE TOOLBOX
CHAPTER 1 **TOOLBOX**

Since Chapter 1 is designed to provide you with a little "Prostate 101" and a few prostate cancer statistics, we don't have the usual worksheets, checklists, or assessment tools to complete. Instead, please use the notes section below to jot down any thoughts or questions you may have.

NOTES:

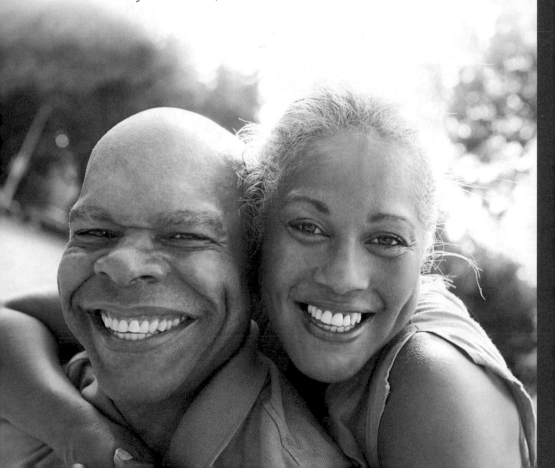

chapter TWO
Do You Need A Prostate Biopsy?

"It's very frightening when you're told you have any form of the C-word, but because of early detection, they caught it before it had hardly begun. I'm completely cured, and will go on to have a wonderful, fruitful life. I'll never die of prostate cancer.

— *Mandy Patinkin, actor*

Patient Story

JOEL

Here's the one thing I want to share with other men like me: If prostate cancer runs in your family, it's very important to get tested — even if you're still young. Just because you're 36 (like I was) doesn't mean you have to wait to get tested. I am glad I pushed it, because they wouldn't have discovered the cancer until it was more advanced.

Five years ago, I went to the doctor to find out about my prostate, because both my dad and my uncle had prostate cancer. I was only 36 years old, and my doctor said I was too young. He said to wait until I was 39.

When I turned 39, my doctor suggested that we wait until I was 40. I told him: 'No, I want run the tests now.' Thank God I did. We caught the cancer very early: Only 1 out of the 24 needles had a small amount of low-risk cancer.

I went to my oldest brother and told him, 'Bro, you should get tested too.' He did, and his biopsy was positive also. He just had CyberKnife treatment, and he's doing fine.

I've been on active surveillance for a year and a half, and I go in for my second MRI next month to see if the cancer is growing. And even if it is, I know I'll get the right treatment.

The second thing I want to share is always get a second opinion — that's what I did.

The first doctors I saw scared the shit out of me. They wanted to cut out my prostate. They said, "Might as well take it out and get it over with." I'm like, wait a minute, I'm only 40 years old. I don't want to wear Pampers for the rest of my life and not be able to have sex.

My uncle lives in Roswell, New Mexico. So he didn't have the same options I do, and 60 percent of his prostate had cancer. He had surgery, and now he leaks when he plays golf, and he still cannot get an erection even though he takes Cialis every day – and he's only 52!

chapter **TWO** summary

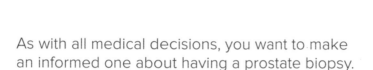

As with all medical decisions, you want to make an informed one about having a prostate biopsy.

Chapter 2 walks you through the test results, images, and information that doctors use when evaluating whether or not a man needs to have a prostate biopsy.

The Prostate Biopsy Assessment Tool in the **Chapter 2 Toolbox** gives you a clear and concise way to use these results, images, and information to better understand why you do (or do not) need a prostate biopsy.

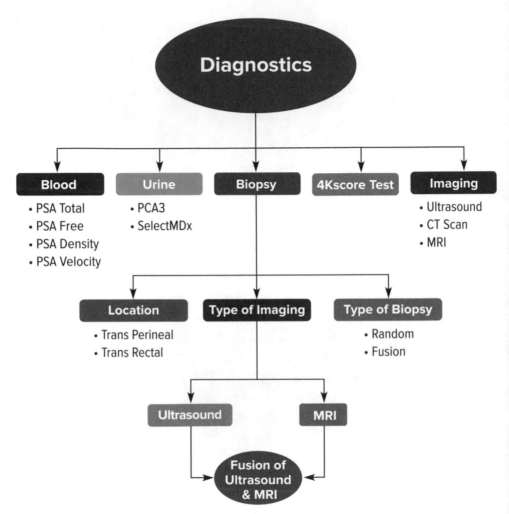

Figure 2.0 outlines the key pieces of information that doctors use to determine whether you have prostate cancer — and how aggressive it is. The **Prostate Biopsy Assessment Tool (Page 56)** in the **Chapter 2 Toolbox** gives you a place to record your own information and put your data in perspective.

DEBUNKING MYTHS

DO PROSTATE BIOPSIES SPREAD CANCER?

The short answer is NO.

After millions of prostate biopsies over many decades, the overwhelming clinical evidence shows nothing to support the idea that prostate cancer spreads along needle tracks after a prostate biopsy.

As Dr. Larry Bans, M.D. of the Cancer Treatment Centers of America puts it, "The risk of 'seeding,' or 'tracking,' or 'spreading' cancer with prostate needle biopsies, if there is a risk at all, has to be exceedingly rare and low."

Currently, prostate biopsies are a necessary part of making an accurate cancer diagnosis. In the near future, however, MRI and other forms of imaging may become so sensitive that biopsies become a thing of the past — or only require a few needles to make the correct diagnosis (instead of today's 12-24 needles).

VOCABULARY

See Glossary for Definitions

4Kscore Test

AUA Score

Benign Prostatic Hyperplasia (BPH)

CAT Scan

ConfirmMDx

Digital Rectal Exam (DRE)

Doppler

Erectile Dysfunction (ED)

Imaging

Lab Tests

Lumbosacral

Magnetic Resonance Imaging (MRI)

Medical History

Needle Cores

PCA3 Urine Test

Pelvic Floor

Prostate Biopsy

Prostatitis

PSA (Prostate Specific Antigen)

PSA Density

PSA Free

PSA Test

PSA Total

PSA Velocity

Sacroiliac

SelectMDx

TRUS (standard) Biopsy

TURP (surgery to relieve BPH)

Ultrasound

Urinary Frequency

Urinary Urgency

NOTE

WHY HAVE A PROSTATE BIOPSY?

Many patients ask, "Why should I have a prostate biopsy? Don't all men develop prostate cancer eventually?" Yes and no. If men live long enough, 1-in-7 will develop some form of clinically significant prostate cancer. Most of these cancers will be low-risk low-volume cancer, which can be treated (at least initially) with active surveillance. Simply stated: There are three main reasons to have a prostate biopsy :

1. *Determine if you have prostate cancer*
2. *If cancer is present, determine which type and how much*
3. *If cancer is present, how life threatening is it?*

PUTTING ALL THE PIECES TOGETHER

There is no simple equation or computer algorithm that tells doctors exactly who needs to have a prostate biopsy — and who does not. However, the following four sources of information, plus your doctor's experience, can help identify patients who may have prostate cancer:

1. Patient history
2. Physical exam
3. Lab tests
4. Imaging

To see how these four sources of information work together, we invite you to use the **Prostate Biopsy Assessment Tool** on **Page 56** in the **Chapter 2 Toolbox.**

These four sources also help rule out conditions such as prostatitis, BPH, and pelvic floor problems, which can all lead to an unnecessary prostate biopsy. (See "The Great Mimickers" on **Page 40**.)

SIGNS THAT YOU MIGHT NEED A PROSTATE BIOPSY

When that familiar, easy feeling of going to the bathroom is replaced by any of the following, it's a good indicator that something is wrong:

- Pain during urination
- Needing to urinate frequently (more than every hour)
- Needing to go NOW!
- Straining to urinate
- Waking up to urinate multiple times at night
- Incomplete emptying of your bladder

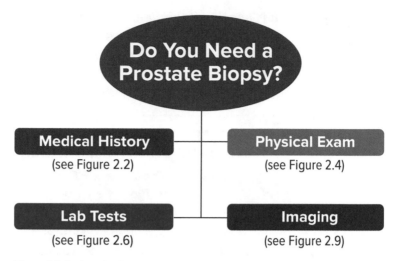

Figure 2.1 displays the four sources of information that doctors frequently use to decide whether a prostate biopsy is the logical next step.

BEFORE YOU HAVE A BIOPSY

If your doctor has already scheduled your prostate biopsy — but has NOT discussed the results from the four sources of information listed in **Figure 2.1** *— we recommend that you make another appointment so you are crystal clear about why your doctor thinks you need a prostate biopsy.*

Why question your doctor's expert opinion? The invention of PSA testing has given rise to a dramatic increase in the number of prostate biopsies performed every year — more than half a million of which are unnecessary. Why expose yourself to unwanted complications from a diagnostic procedure that you don't actually need?

Sometimes it helps to have a second opinion to answer your questions and address your doubts — and see if a prostate biopsy is the best course of action.

THE GREAT MIMICKERS

It is important to rule out prostate cancer mimickers like BPH and prostatitis before you have a prostate biopsy; however, a prostate biopsy is well worth the risk to dismiss the possibility of advanced prostate cancer.

THERE ARE TWO COMMON CONDITIONS THAT MIMIC PROSTATE CANCER:

1. **Enlarged Prostate** *or* **BPH**
   (Benign Prostatic Hyperplasia)
2. **Prostatitis** *(pain, itching, swelling, of the prostate and/or nearby tissue)*

Both of these conditions can cause symptoms similar to those of advanced prostate cancer. All three raise your PSA levels. (Early prostate cancer rarely has symptoms.)

BPH *is a non-cancerous growth of the prostate that occurs in most men as they age. Approximately half of American men over 50 have some symptoms related to BPH.*

Prostatitis *(prostate inflammation or infection) is often called, "a headache in the pelvis." More than two million American men visit their doctor every year with prostatitis.*

There are four kinds of prostatitis, but 95 percent of cases fall into the "Chronic Nonbacterial" category, which means the symptoms have been going on for months (sometimes years) and they aren't being caused by a detectable bacterial infection.

Both an enlarged prostate and prostatitis can cause symptoms that are similar to advanced prostate cancer:

- *Low flow (weak urinary stream)*
- *Having to push to drain your bladder*
- *Urinary urgency (gotta go NOW!)*
- *Urinary frequency (the need to go every hour)*
- *Waking up to pee in the middle of the night (nocturia)*
- *Painful urination (dysuria)*
- *Itching, burning, or pain in the prostate area*

1. MEDICAL HISTORY

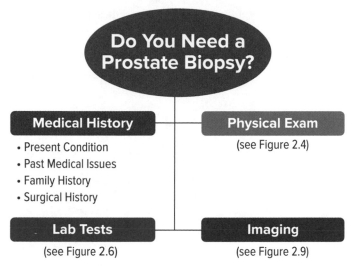

Figure 2.2 outlines the items in a medical history that can tip the scales one way or the other about having a prostate biopsy.

PRESENT CONDITION

Urinary symptoms are seldom present in men with early stage prostate cancer. If you are having urinary symptoms like those listed on **Page 40**, there is very a high probability that BPH, prostatitis, or advanced prostate cancer is the culprit.

Unfortunately, by the time prostate cancer has advanced enough to cause urinary symptoms, 95 percent of those men have prostate cancer outside their prostate (metastatic disease). Prostate cancer is much easier to treat when it is still inside the prostate (local disease).

Fortunately, BPH and prostatitis are the most common causes of urinary symptoms.

For example, if your urinary problems have steadily increased for a few years, an enlarged prostate is the likely cause.

Likewise, prostatitis can create the urgent need to go to the bathroom RIGHT NOW or feeling like you have to go every-hour-on-the-hour. Prostatitis can also create pain and itching that wanders up and down the urethra or extends up into the bladder.

If you're having urination issues, we encourage you take the American Urological Association (AUA) questionnaire (See **Page 63**), and go over it with your doctor.

According to the American Cancer Society, the 5-year survival rate for treating **all stages** of prostate cancer is 99 percent, which includes the survival rates for cancers that have spread outside the prostate but are still within the pelvis ("regional" metastatic disease).

The 5-year survival rate for treating prostate cancer that has spread to distant lymph nodes, organs, and bones throughout the body ("distant"metastatic disease), sadly, is only 28 percent.

Ruling out distant metastatic disease is why it is so important to let your doctor know if you've every had any of the following:

- BPH
- Prostatitis
- Urinary Tract Infections (UTIs)
- Urinary strictures (scarring inside the urethra that prevents the normal flow of urine)
- A serious car accident (or other injury) that caused significant trauma to your lower back, pelvis, hips, or lower extremities?
- Other major diseases such as diabetes, heart disease, stroke, autoimmune disorders, COPD, asthma, or other cancers ... to name just a few.

Although this is only a partial list (a full list would take pages), these **past medical issues** provide your doctor with important clues about what's causing your prostate problems: cancer or other "easier to treat" conditions.

Bottom line: Talk to your healthcare providers. Give them all the information they need about your past and present conditions and injuries. This information will help them determine whether you are a good candidate for a prostate biopsy.

Also, list all the medications you are currently taking and all the medications you've been prescribed in the past year. This information is essential so your medical team can create a comprehensive prostate snapshot.

FAMILY HISTORY

Prostate cancer runs in families.

A man who has a father or brother who developed

prostate cancer is two times more likely to develop this disease. The chances go up if prostate cancer was detected before the age 55, or if three or more family members develop prostate cancer. The risk of developing prostate cancer is slightly higher if a brother had the disease than if a father did.

Also, men from families in which the women have had breast or ovarian cancer are at a higher risk of developing prostate cancer.

SURGICAL HISTORY

Previous surgeries affect the outcomes of future prostate cancer treatments. For example, if you have had a TURP (TransUrethral Resection of the Prostate) for an enlarged prostate, you may be at a higher risk for incontinence, which could impact your decision process.

Your surgical history is also important because even the most successful surgeries leave scar tissue behind that can make a biopsy or additional surgery more difficult.

Surgeries (or injuries) to other areas of your body can also impact the health of your prostate. For example, a surgery that has a long-term affect on how you walk, run, stand, or sit can eventually impact the health of your pelvic floor (also called your "urinary sphincter").

Essentially, anything that has a negative effect on the overall health of your pelvis will probably cause problems for your prostate, too. If you've had any surgeries, it's important to tell your doctor about them.

LABORATORY (LAB) TESTS

Blood tests like PSA (free and total), comparisons like PSA Velocity and PSA Density, and urine tests such as PCA3 and SelectMDx help identify men who are more likely to have prostate cancer.

Newer tests such as SelectMDx and 4Kscore Test help identify men who have a higher risk of developing aggressive prostate cancer.

These tests support a doctor's decision to recommend that a patient have a prostate biopsy or to wait for a period of time (usually between three months and a year) to repeat the tests.

Risk Factors	Information	Comments
Age	• Median age of diagnosis is 66. • 6 in 10 men are diagnosed after 65. • African American should start screening after age 40.	Your health history and family health history of longevity are important factors.
Race (Death Rates per 100,000)	• African American 47.2 • Native American 20.2 • White 19.9 • Hispanic 17.8 • Asian/Pacific Islander 9.4	Race can help doctors decide who should have a biopsy and at what age. African American men and native Hawaiian men do not have the same cancer risk, even if they are the same age and have the same test results.
Present Illness	• Includes suspicious signs/symptoms of advanced prostate cancer • Results of previous lab tests, imaging, and diagnostic tests are important baseline information.	Severity, duration, and timing of symptoms help rule out conditions that can mimic prostate cancer (BPH & prostatitis).
Past Medical	Identify other medical conditions that could increase complication rates and/or limit your survival.	These medical conditions include diabetes, heart disease, stroke, neurogenic bladder, lumbar disc disease, other cancers, and so on.
Urologic	• Previous urologic surgeries • History of urethral stricture • Presence of prostatitis or BPH • History or presence of stones in the kidneys, bladder, or prostate	Certain urologic conditions should be addressed before prostate cancer treatment, as they may limit the type of treatment or hamper recovery from treatment.
Surgical	• Previous abdominal or pelvic surgeries can affect your structure or create scar tissue that limits proposed treatment(s) • Previous orthopedic surgeries can affect function of the urinary sphincter and bladder	Previous surgeries, spinal injuries, or orthopedic injuries may increase prostate cancer treatment complication rates and may limit future treatment choices.
Family	Your prostate cancer risk is 2-5 times higher if your father and/or brother has prostate cancer before age 65.	Your prostate cancer risk also rises if your mother and/or sister have had breast or cervical cancer
Social (Habits)	Smoking, chronic/binge drinking, recreational drug use, or prescription drug abuse may affect your general health, liver function, and immune system.	You need to be honest with all your healthcare providers about your vices/addictions; otherwise, there could be severe complications from treatment.

Figure 2.3 lists the risk factors that can influence the decision to have a prostate biopsy. (See **Page 56**.)

2. PHYSICAL EXAM

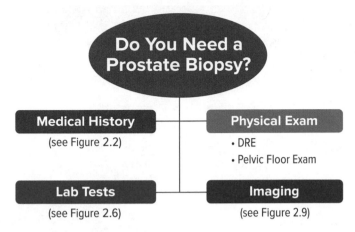

Do You Need a Prostate Biopsy?

Medical History
(see Figure 2.2)

Physical Exam
• DRE
• Pelvic Floor Exam

Lab Tests
(see Figure 2.6)

Imaging
(see Figure 2.9)

Figure 2.4 lists the two physical exams that you should receive during your evaluation for a prostate biopsy: DRE and Pelvic Floor Exam. These tests are normally done at the same time.

WHAT IS A DIGITAL RECTAL EXAM (DRE)?

A DRE is a physical exam where your doctor inserts a lubricated, gloved finger (digit) into your rectum and checks for any prostate irregularities that can be felt through the wall of the rectum. These irregularities include:

- Asymmetry (the two sides of your prostate should feel the same)
- Size (big, little, average)
- Texture (soft, hard, or both in different places)
- Lumps and bumps that could indicate cancer

A DRE can also help identify or rule out prostate cancer mimickers like prostatitis, enlarged prostate, and problems caused by lopsided tension on your urinary sphincter (pelvic floor dysfunction). Wait 48 hours between a DRE and PSA test.

WHAT IS THE DIFFERENCE BETWEEN A DRE AND A PELVIC FLOOR EXAMINATION?

Most doctors perform a digital rectal exam of the prostate and a pelvic floor examination at the same time. A DRE gives doctors all the prostate information listed above, and a pelvic floor exam allows doctors to feel for areas of rigid and relaxed muscles. Tight, loose, or uneven muscular tone in the pelvic floor/urinary sphincter indicates a high probability of a structural component to your prostate problems.

	If/Then	Comments
DRE *(Normal)*	**If PSA 2-4:** 15% risk of positive biopsy **If PSA 4-10:** 25% risk of positive biopsy **If PSA >10:** 50% risk of positive biopsy	• Highly subjective • Operator dependent • Urologist is generally more accurate than a single blood test
DRE *(Abnormal)*	**If PSA 2-4:** 20% risk of positive biopsy **If PSA 4-10:** 45% risk of positive biopsy **If PSA >10:** 75% risk of positive biopsy	

Figure 2.5 illustrates the connection between digital rectal exams (DRE), PSA, and the risk of having a positive prostate biopsy.

---

3. LAB TESTS

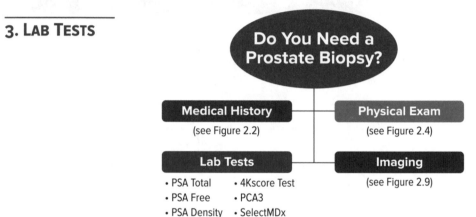

Figure 2.6 lists the lab tests that are most likely to indicate the presence of prostate cancer; therefore, suggesting that a prostate biopsy is the next logical step.

The easiest way to classify **Lab Tests** is look at which body fluid is being tested:

BLOOD

- **PSA (free & total):** The lower the PSA Total number and the higher the PSA Free number, the better.
- **PSA Density:** Considers prostate size with PSA total: the bigger the prostate, the higher the PSA.
- **PSA Velocity:** How your PSA Total numbers change over time.
- **Hormone Levels:** (recommended) Total testosterone, free testosterone, total estrogen, and testosterone/ estrogen ratio.
- **4Kscore Test:** Combines 4 blood biomarkers with age, DRE result, and biopsy results (if any) to assess the probability of finding aggressive prostate cancer.

Lab Test: Blood	
Information	**Comments**
PSA Total **Normal Ranges for Adult Men** • 0.0-2.5 in 40-49 year olds. • 2.6-3.5 in 50-59 year olds. • 3.6-4.5 in 60-69 year olds. • 4.6-6.5 in 70-79 year olds.	• Increased by: BPH, infection, inflammation, ejaculation, prostatic massage, riding bicycles, DRE, TRUS, prostate biopsy, and cystoscopy. • Decreased by: certain herbs, medications, and products that contain estrogen. • PSA can vary by 3.6% from day to day • Still the best first alert system
PSA Free • Free PSA is an unbound form of PSA released by BPH cells • Helpful when PSA is between 4-10 • If free PSA > 25%, the likely culprit for an elevated PSA is an enlarged prostate (BPH)	• If free PSA is between 0-10%: there is a 56% chance prostate cancer • 10-15%: there is a 28% chance prostate cancer • 15-20%: there is a 20% chance prostate cancer • 20-25%: there is a 16% chance prostate cancer • >25%: there is an 8% chance prostate cancer
PSA Density • PSA Density is a ratio of PSA to prostate size (See **Page 54**). • It is calculated by dividing PSA by the volume of prostate, calculated by ultrasound or MRI. • You need a TRUS or MRI to determine PSA Density (a DRE not accurate enough).	• A PSA Density of less than 0.07 is likely to be caused by BPH. • 0.07-0.15: Uncertain. • A PSA Density of greater than 0.15 is suspicious for prostate cancer.
PSA Velocity • Measures the rate of change over time • Requires 3 PSA tests within a 2- year period	• A PSA velocity increase of 0.75 ng/ml per year, or an increase of more than 20% per year is suspicious for prostate cancer. • You need to rule out: BPH, infection, inflammation, ejaculation, prostatic massage, riding bicycles, DRE, previous biopsies & cystoscopy.
4Kscore Test • 4 kallikrein levels: PSA Total, PSA Free, PSA Intact, and hK2 • Also takes age, DRE, and prior biopsy results into account • Algorithm calculates risk of aggressive prostate cancer	• Tests like PSA and PCA3 are used to assess a man's risk of having prostate cancer; whereas the 4Kscore Test identifies a man's risk of having *aggressive* prostate cancer. • A reliable indicator that accurately identifies aggressive (high-risk) prostate cancer.

Figure 2.7 explains the various values to watch for with blood tests. Please see the **Prostate Biopsy Assessment Tool (Page 56)** in the **Chapter 2 Toolbox** to include your own information.

URINE

- **PCA3:** This test reveals a gene that is highly expressed in prostate cancer cells. Unlike PSA, PCA3 is NOT affected by an enlarged prostate (BPH) or inflammation (prostatitis). A positive PCA3 test is a strong indicator of prostate cancer.

- **SelectMDx:** This test helps identify men who have a higher risk of developing aggressive prostate cancer. It also accurately predicts whether a biopsy will find low-grade or high-grade cancer.

Lab Test: Urine		
PCA 3	• Non-invasive urine-based, molecular test. • Uses the first part of the urine stream after a DRE & prostate massage. • Measures Prostate Cancer Antigen 3 (PCA3): a gene only present in the prostate and highly expressed in prostate cancer.	• PCA3 is unchanged by BPH, infection, inflammation, ejaculation, prostatic massage, riding bicycles, DRE, or previous prostate biopsies. • If positive, IDs patients who need a prostate biopsy, despite previous negative biopsies. • A high PCA3 Score indicates a greater need for a positive biopsy. • A low PCA3 Score indicates a decreased need for a positive biopsy.
SelectMDx	• Non-invasive urine-based, molecular test. • Uses first part of the urine stream after DRE and prostate massage • Measures the expression of DLX1 and HOXC6 genes. Both are associated with an increased probability for high grade prostate cancer (Gleason Score ≥ 7)	• Helps ID men with a higher risk for aggressive prostate cancer. • Accurately predicts the likelihood of finding low-grade & high-grade cancer in a biopsy • Helps determine which patients need a follow-up biopsy right away. • Reduces the need for unnecessary biopsies & other costly tests for men who have a low risk for having prostate cancer.

Figure 2.8 Lists the two main state-of-the-art urine tests that doctors use to evaluate whether a man should have a prostate biopsy or wait for another round of tests. See **Page 57** to include your own information.

The following imaging studies give your medical team more information about your prostate:

1. Doppler Ultrasound (also measures blood flow)
2. CAT scan
3. MRI
4. MRIS (MRI plus spectroscopy that includes info about cellular activity and metabolism)
5. MRI Fusion (Layers an MRI on top of an ultrasound image to create a 3-D view of the prostate)

4. IMAGING

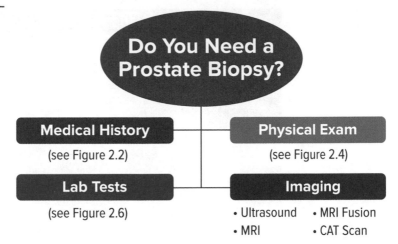

Figure 2.9 lists the main images doctors use to evaluate the health of your prostate.

Both MRI and a CAT scans are used throughout the country in prostate imaging. Image quality and modalities vary from region to region.

How do you know whether to have an MRI or a CAT scan of your prostate? That's a tough call. We recommend you talk to your doctor(s) and any local prostate cancer support groups and find out which imaging facility in your area provides the best results.

Imaging technology has come a long way in the last decade, but it has not evolved to the point where your doctor can tell whether or not you have cancer or how aggressive the cancer is.

For that, you still need a biopsy.

The **Prostate Biopsy Assessment Tool (Page 56)** in the **Chapter 2 Toolbox** gives you a way to look at your test results and image information like a doctor would.

Obviously, a bunch of numbers on a page cannot replace the one-on-one interactions you have with your doctor; however, understanding why a prostate biopsy is (or is not) your logical next step is important.

Understanding leads to knowledge, and knowledge gives you the tools you need to make informed decisions about having a biopsy and your health in general.

We encourage you to take advantage of the tools in the **Chapter 2 Toolbox,** because if you have prostate cancer, it's better to know *now* than *later*.

TYPES OF BIOPSIES

Biopsies	Rectal	Perineal
The Numbers	• Rectal Bleeding: 50% • Infection Rates: 15.5% • Positive Biopsy Rate: 48% • Perineal swelling: 3% • Less painful	• Rectal Bleeding: 3.4% • Infection Rate: 3.4% • Positive Biopsy Rate: 44% • Perineal swelling: 14% • More painful

Figure 2.10 lists the pros and cons of rectal and perineal prostate biopsies. Urinary tract symptoms, pain/difficulty urinating, and urinary retention rates are the same for both kinds of biopsies; however, rectal bleeding, infection, perineal swelling rates, and post-procedure pain are not. Unless there is a compelling medical reason not to, we recommend that you go with the type of biopsy your urologist performs regularly. Frequency is the key here: The more frequently your doctor performs a particular type of biopsy, the better he/she is at doing that procedure.

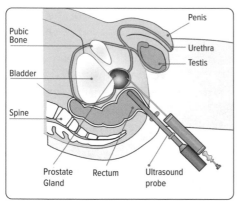

Rectal Prostate Biopsy

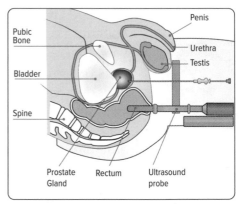

Perineal Prostate Biopsy

Figure 2.11 displays the differences between the two kinds of prostate biopsies: Rectal and Perineal.

A WORD ABOUT MRI FUSION PROSTATE BIOPSIES

The combination of an MRI with an ultrasound image significantly improves the accuracy of a prostate biopsy, and decreases the number of biopsies needed to determine if prostate cancer is present. An MRI fusion biopsy is 70-75% accurate in diagnosing existing prostate cancer versus 30-35% for a TRUS/random biopsy. MRI fusion technology is a significant step in decreasing unnecessary biopsies, and cuts down on the number of core samples obtained during a biopsy; therefore, minimizing complications. (Higher accuracy leads to fewer biopsies; fewer biopsy needles leads to fewer complications).

ADVANTAGES AND DISADVANTAGES OF THE THREE MOST COMMON TYPES OF PROSTATE BIOPSIES

	Advantages	Disadvantages
TRUS / Random	• TRUS is relatively inexpensive • The ultrasound determines the size and shape of the prostate, suggest areas of cancer, calcifications, and blood flow • Most urologists use ultrasound equipment in their office • All urologists train with TRUS • TRUS is an evenly spaced "random" needle biopsy that uses a total of 12-24 needles, depending on the size of the prostate.	• TRUS does not detect all cancer areas. • TRUS is considered random in most cases • Quality of the ultrasound equipment is crucial in the improved detection of suspicious areas. • Doppler can be helpful in identifying more suspicious areas • The risk of infection and trauma to rectal wall goes up with the number of biopsies • TRUS can miss up to 70% of cancers on the first biopsy
MRI / Guided	• Very high resolution of suspicious areas • Decreased number of needles, minimizing trauma to rectal wall; thus, reducing the risk of infection • Important for creating a baseline for future MRI monitoring • Helpful in active surveillance patients • Helpful in staging as it can detect extracapsular extension and seminal vesicle involvement • Can detect lymph node involvement and/or bone involvement	• Expensive procedure • Claustrophobic patients may need medication to manage anxiety • Quality of the MRI technology varies • Few physicians are properly trained in the use of this technology
MRI Fusion	• Increased detection of high-risk prostate cancer • Decreased detection of low-risk prostate cancer • Radiologists experienced in reading and interpreting MRI images are essential in mapping the abnormal areas	• Fusion images are susceptible to a patient's movement resulting in imprecise segmentation of the gland outline and decreased accuracy • Doctors must learn to read MRI images • Additional time is required for the image segmentation and matching processes • MRI Fusion can miss up to 30% of cancers on the first biopsy

Figure 2.12 outlines the advantages and disadvantages of the different types of prostate biopsies.

Doctor Story
DR. KURT STROM, MD

Urology,
Banner Health
Loveland, Colorado

As a medical student, I remember the chairman of Rush University Medical Center proclaiming that sometime in the near future there would be a pill that cures prostate cancer. While that "magic pill" still eludes us, I marvel at how far prostate cancer treatment of has come during my brief career.

Back in 2007, as a resident performing open radical prostatectomies, I watched skilled surgeons lose copious amounts of blood. Halfway through my training, our hospital bought a DaVinci S surgical robot, and I witnessed seasoned urologists struggle to become skilled robotic surgeons.

Despite the cost of the robot (millions of dollars), the blood loss was minimal, patients went home the next day and back to work within a week. These improvements in care were hugely important to my patients and their families — parts of the healthcare equation that economists cannot assign a dollar value.

In May 2012, the United States Preventative Services Task Force (USPSTF) stated that PSA screening for prostate cancer was inappropriately overused. Doctors could do little but watch as prostate cancer treatment rates fell dramatically. It was a conspiracy against men.

Despite how wrongheaded this decision was, it challenged urologists to rethink how to better treat men with prostate cancer — and men who may develop it.

For example, we have stopped treating non-lethal low-risk prostate cancer, because the unwanted complications of treatment often outweigh the benefits. It's changes like this that keep me hopeful that prostate cancer treatment is moving in the right direction.

LOOKING AHEAD

CHAPTER 1: You or your doctor is concerned about your prostate — We provide you with **Prostate 101**: where it lives, what it does, plus relevant statistics.

CHAPTER 2: Your doctor told you to **schedule a prostate biopsy** — We give you a **Prostate Biopsy Assessment Tool** to see if you actually need one, and what to expect if you do.

CHAPTER 3: You have a prostate biopsy — We explain the steps you need to take, whether you have a **negative biopsy or a positive biopsy**.

CHAPTER 4: You want to **use your cancer diagnosis as a springboard to better health** — We help you address your wellness goals with a proven plan that covers inflammation, diet, inactivity, stress, immune system, hormones, structure, and removing toxic substances.

WHAT'S NEXT?

I Had a Prostate Biopsy
Go To Chapter 3

I Had a Positive Biopsy
Get a Second Opinion

I Need Help with My Overall Health & Wellness
Go To Chapter 4

I Need More Information
Read
Prostate Cancer: A New Approach...

WELCOME TO THE TOOLBOX
CHAPTER 2 **TOOLBOX**

THIS TOOLBOX SECTION INCLUDES THE FOLLOWING TOOLS AND RESOURCES TO HELP YOU MAKE AN INFORMED DECISION ABOUT HAVING A PROSTATE BIOPSY:

- PSA Density Calculator
- Prostate Cancer Risk Factors
- Prostate Biopsy Assessment Tool
- Frequently Asked Questions
- How to Prepare for an Outpatient Prostate Biopsy Procedure
- Post-biopsy Instructions
- A Word about Blood Thinners
- AUA Score

The information that you provide in the "Your Data" column of the next three tables helps clarify your decision to have (or not to have) a prostate biopsy.

PSA Density Calculator

	HOW TO CALCULATE	YOUR DATA
Prostate Volume	• The easiest way to calculate your Prostate Volume is with a trans-rectal ultrasound image that measures the length, width, and height of the prostate (prostate volume). • Once you have these numbers, multiply them together (L x W x H), then multiply that number by 0.52	**You have to know your Prostate Volume to calculate your PSA Density.**
PSA Density	• Calculate your Prostate Volume with either a trans-rectal ultrasound, MRI, or CT scan. • Divide your PSA Total number by your total Prostate Volume to find the PSA Density. • For example, if you have a PSA Total of 4.0 ng/ml and a prostate volume of 30 ml, divide 4.0 by 30. $$4.0 \div 30 = 0.15$$	• **Less than 0.07 = likely BPH** • **0.07-0.15 = uncertain** • **More than 0.15 = suspicious for prostate cancer**

Prostate Cancer Risk Factors

	INFORMATION	COMMENTS	YOUR DATA
AGE	• If older than 75, no need for screening • If you have a family history of cancer or are African American, start screening at age 40	• Not an exact science. • Your health history is very important • History of longevity in your family is also important	**Your Age**
RACE *(Death rates per 100,000)*	• African American 47.2 • Native American 20.2 • White 19.9 • Hispanic 17.8 • Asian/Pacific Islander 9.4	Knowing your racial identity can help determine when you should have your first prostate biopsy	**Ethnicity**
MEDICAL HISTORY	Do you have any medical conditions that could limit your 5-year survival?	Do you have any medical conditions that could increase complications rates of prostate cancer treatments?	**Medical History**
FAMILY HISTORY	If you are under 65 years old and either your father, brother, or both had prostate cancer, then your risk of developing prostate cancer is 2-5 times higher.	If your mother and/or sister had breast or cervical cancer, then your chances of having prostate cancer also increases.	**Cancer History**
If Digital Rectal Exam is Normal	• If PSA 2-4, 15% probability of positive biopsy • If PSA 4-10, 25% probability of positive biopsy • PSA >10, 50% probability of positive biopsy	• Highly subjective • Operator-dependent • DREs performed by urologists are generally more accurate	**PSA w/ Normal DRE**
If Digital Rectal Exam is Abnormal	• PSA 2-4, 20% probability of positive biopsy • PSA 4-10, 45% probability of positive biopsy • PSA >10, 75% probability of positive biopsy	• Highly subjective • Operator-dependent • DREs performed by urologists are generally more accurate	**PSA w/ Abnormal DRE**

TOOLBOX

Prostate Biopsy Assessment Tool

	INFORMATION	COMMENTS	YOUR DATA
PSA Total	**Normal Total PSA Range** • 0.0-2.5 in 40-49 year olds • 2.6-3.5 in 50-59 year olds • 3.6-4.5 in 60-69 year olds • 4.6-6.5 in 70-79 year olds • Still the best first alert system • Like a "Check Engine" light on your car's dashboard	• Increased by: BPH, infection, inflammation, ejaculation, prostatic massage, riding bicycles, DRE, TRUS, prostate biopsy, and cystoscopy. • **Decreased by:** certain herbs, medications such as 5 alpha reductase inhibitors, and products that contain estrogen. • PSA can vary by 3.6% from day to day	**Total PSA?**
PSA Free	• Free PSA is an unbound form of PSA released by BPH cells • Helpful when PSA is between 4-10 • If free PSA is greater than 25%, the likely culprit for an elevated PSA is an enlarged prostate (BPH).	• If free PSA is between 0-10%, there is a 56% chance of prostate cancer • 10-15%, there is a 28% chance of prostate cancer • 15-20%, there is a 20% chance of prostate cancer • 20-25%, there is a 16% chance of prostate cancer • More than 25% there is an 8% chance of prostate cancer	**Free PSA?**
PSA Density	• PSA Density is a ratio of PSA to prostate size. • It is calculated by dividing PSA Total by the volume of prostate (calculated by ultrasound or MRI) • You need TRUS or MRI to determine density (DRE not reliable)	• A PSA Density of less than 0.07 is likely to be caused by BPH • 0.07-0.15: Uncertain • Greater than 0.15: Suspicious for prostate cancer	**PSA Density?** *(See Page 54)*
PSA Velocity	Requires 3 PSA tests in a 2-year period	• A PSA velocity increase of 0.75 ng/ml per year, or an increase of more than 20% per year is suspicious for prostate cancer. • You need to rule out: BPH, infection, inflammation, ejaculation, prostatic massage, riding bicycles, DRE, previous biopsies, and cystoscopy.	**PSA Velocity?**

TOOLBOX

Prostate Biopsy Assessment Tool Cont.

	INFORMATION	COMMENTS	YOUR DATA
4Kscore Test	• 4 kallikrein levels: Total PSA, Free PSA, intact PSA and hK2 • Includes age, DRE, and prior biopsy status • Algorithm calculates risk of aggressive prostate cancer	• Highly sensitive test that is a clear indicator of aggressive prostate cancer • The only blood test that accurately identifies risk for aggressive prostate cancer	**4Kscore Test**
PCA3	• Non-invasive urine-based molecular test • Uses first part of the urine stream after DRE and prostate massage • If you have a positive PCA-3 test and a negative biopsy, a 2nd biopsy is encouraged because of the high likelihood of having prostate cancer.	PCA-3 is not changed by BPH, infection, inflammation, ejaculation, prostatic massage, riding bicycles, DRE, previous prostate biopsies, or cystoscopy.	**PCA3 Score**
SelectMDx	• Non-invasive urine-based molecular test • Uses first part of the urine stream after DRE and prostate massage • Measures the expression of DLX1 and HOXC6 genes. Both are associated with an increased probability for high-grade prostate cancer (Gleason Score ≥ 7)	• Helps ID men with a higher risk for aggressive prostate cancer • Can accurately predict the likelihood of finding low-grade & high-grade cancer in a biopsy • Helps determine which patients need a follow-up biopsy sooner • Reduces the need for unnecessary biopsies & other costly tests for men who have a low risk of having prostate cancer	**SelectMDx**

TOOLBOX

Frequently Asked Questions about Ultrasound-Guided Transrectal Needle Biopsy of Prostate

---

TOP 6 QUESTIONS THAT PATIENTS ASK ABOUT PROSTATE BIOPSIES:

1. Why should I have a prostate biopsy?
2. What do I need to do before I have one?
3. What are the possible side effects of a prostate biopsy?
4. Will it hurt?
5. What if my prostate biopsy comes back positive?
6. Why do I need a biopsy if MRI imaging suggests I have prostate cancer?

---

1. Why should I have a prostate biopsy?

When doctors recommend that their patients have a prostate biopsy, they are attempting to do two things:

1. Rule out the presence of prostate cancer
2. If prostate cancer is present, determine type, stage, Gleason Score, and the extent of the cancer.

The earlier you catch prostate cancer, the easier it is to cure. If prostate cancer is present, it's better to know sooner than later.

2. What do I need to do before I have one?

The logistics of a prostate biopsy are fairly straightforward:

BEFORE THE PROCEDURE

- You will be asked to use a Fleet enema at home two hours before the procedure.
- You will be given some oral antibiotics to take as a precaution against infection from the procedure.

DURING THE PROCEDURE

- The procedure is usually done in your doctor's office.
- It usually takes 20-30 minutes.
- Unless you require anti-anxiety medication, you can drive yourself home.
- A lubricated ultrasound probe is inserted into your rectum. This probe also doubles as the guide for the biopsy needles.

- Between 12-24 needles will be used to extract a small amount of tissue from your prostate, which will be analyzed and evaluated by a pathologist (a doctor who specializes in tissue analysis).

AFTER THE PROCEDURE

- You will be given additional antibiotics after the procedure.
- It takes about a week to get the results back.
- It is normal to pee and ejaculate blood for up to two weeks. The blood will be bright red at first and then fade to brown before it goes a way completely.
- If you have persistent pain or inflammation in your prostate (like you have a tennis ball between your legs), fever, flu-like symptoms, muscle aches, or your body starts to shake uncontrollably, go to the nearest emergency room or urgent care center. These are all symptoms of sepsis (a systemic blood infection), a rare but potentially fatal side effect of a prostate biopsy.

3. What are the possible side effects of a prostate biopsy?

All surgical procedures, including prostate biopsies, carry some risk of side effects:

- Infection — which can be fatal in a very low percentage of cases (1 to 3 men per 1,000)
- Prostatitis (itching, scratching, and pain in the prostate and/or urethra)
- Difficulty urinating
- Urinary frequency (the urge to pee frequently)
- Urinary Urgency (gotta go RIGHT NOW!)
- Temporary ED
- Blood in your urine
- Blood in your semen
- Lingering pain

These side effects usually go away on their own. They may increase in number and severity after repeated biopsies (2nd, 3rd ...).

TOOLBOX

4. Will it hurt?

When we explain the above information to most men, they nod their heads "yes" at all the right moments, but when we ask them if they have any questions, the first one they ask is, "Will it hurt?"

When the injection of a local anesthetic is done correctly, which happens 99% of the time, the pain of a prostate biopsy is low (1 or 2 out of 10, with 10 being the worst pain you've ever felt). If the anesthetic injection is done incorrectly, a prostate biopsy feels like what it is — a bunch of needles being shot through the wall of your rectum and into your prostate (8 out of 10 pain).

Hint: Ask the doctor to make sure that you are "totally numb" before the first biopsy needle.

5. What if my prostate biopsy comes back positive?

The point of this book is to help men (and their loved ones) understand all the factors that go into (or should go into) the decision to have a prostate biopsy.

If your prostate biopsy finds any amount of prostate cancer, we recommend that you buy a copy of **Prostate Cancer: A New Approach to Diagnosis, Treatment, and Health** or ask your doctor to provide one for you.

6. Why do I need a biopsy if MRI imaging suggests I have prostate cancer?

Imaging technology has come a long way in the last decade. That said, MRI technology has not advanced to the point where it can tell you whether or not you have cancer, or more importantly, how aggressive the cancer is. Doctors still need a "tissue diagnosis" to do that.

Preparation for an Outpatient Prostate Biopsy

The following information expands upon our answers to the previous six questions. We include this information because our experience tells us that different patients need to hear the same information presented in different ways before they "get it."

This procedure is usually done in your urologist's office and involves firing and retracting several needles (12 to 24) into the prostate to retrieve small samples of tissue. A real-time ultrasound image is used to guide the needles, and the procedure usually takes between 20 to 30 minutes, depending upon the number of needles.

Standard suggestions include:

- Consume only clear liquids the day of the procedure.
- Use a Fleet enema the morning of the procedure to clear stool from the rectum. **This is very important!** A Fleet enema can be purchased at any drugstore,
- You may be given 2 prescriptions, as well as some anti-anxiety medication just before the biopsy.
- Come to the procedure with your bladder at least partially full of urine (at least one hour without urinating).
- You can go home after the biopsy. Please continue to take the antibiotics until all the pills are gone.
- Please continue to take your other medications (except blood thinners) that you are taking under the direction of your physician(s).

You may experience the following problems after the biopsy:

- Bleeding from the rectum
- Blood in your urine and semen — a common and disconcerting problem that usually lasts 2-3 weeks.
- Mild burning, pain, or increased need to urinate — these symptoms are not a concern unless they persist for more than 24 hours.

If you develop fever, chills, flu-like symptoms, the pain increases, or you cannot urinate — **let your doctor know immediately!**

Post Trans Rectal Ultrasound and Prostate Biopsy Instructions

It is extremely important that you finish your antibiotics. Also, increase your fluid intake for the first two days after the biopsy to decrease formation of blood clots in your urine. Usually, your urine will clear itself of blood clots after the first few times you pee. Blood spotting in your urine may occur for up to a week.

TOOLBOX

Your rectum or the base of your penis may hurt for a couple of days. That's normal.

Staying off your feet until the morning after your biopsy is a good idea. Limit your activity, particularly heavy lifting, for 48 hours or until the bleeding stops. Avoid cycling for one week.

IT IS IMPORTANT TO CONTACT YOUR DOCTOR IMMEDIATELY (OR GO TO YOUR LOCAL EMERGENCY ROOM) IF ANY OF THE FOLLOWING SYMPTOMS OCCUR:

- Sharp pain or intense burning while urinating
- Chills
- Fever
- Excessive blood clots or lots of blood in the urine or stool
- Difficulty or inability to urinate
- Overall weakness or feeling like you're going to faint

A Word or Two about Blood Thinners

Talk to your doctor(s) about ALL the medications you are taking: prescription, over-the-counter, nutritional supplements, and so on.

We recommend that you bring all the bottles and containers to show your doctor(s) — **BEFORE YOU HAVE A PROSTATE BIOPSY.**

If you don't want to carry all those bottles with you to your next appointment, write down a complete list of all the pills, powders, potions, and lotions you use.

The reason we want you to show your doctor(s) the medications and supplements you take is because some of them may contain blood-thinning compounds.

Avoiding blood thinners is one of the most important things you can do to ensure that you have a successful prostate biopsy.

Again, talk to your doctor(s). They will be happy to clarify what you shouldn't take before your biopsy.

Your **AUA** score gives you and your doctors a way to quantify your urinary symptoms. If you haven't filled out an **AUA** score recently, take a minute to do so, and share the results with your doctors.

AUA Symptom Score (AUASS)

Circle One Number on Each Line	Not at All	Less Than 1 Time in 5	Less Than Half the Time	About Half The Time	More Than Half The Time	Almost Always
Over the past month, how often have you had the feeling of not completely emptying your bladder after you finished urinating?	0	1	2	3	4	5
Over the past month, how often have you had to urinate again less than 2 hours after you finished urinating?	0	1	2	3	4	5
Over the past month, how often have you found that you stopped and started again several times when you urinated?	0	1	2	3	4	5
Over the past month, how often have you found it hard to hold your urine?	0	1	2	3	4	5
Over the past month, how often have you had a weak urine stream?	0	1	2	3	4	5
Over the past month, how often have you had to push or strain to begin urination?	0	1	2	3	4	5
	None	1 Time	2 Times	3 Times	4 Times	5 or More Times
Over the past month, how many times per night did you most typically get up to urinate from the time you went to bed at night until the time you got up in the morning?	0	1	2	3	4	5

Add the score for each number above and write the total in the space to the right _____

SYMPTOM SCORE: 1-7 (Mild) 8-19 (Moderate) 20-35 (Severe)

Quality of Life (QOL)

Circle One Number on Each Line	Delighted	Pleased	Mostly Satisfied	Mixed	Mostly Dis-satisfied	Unhappy	Terrible
How would you feel if you had to live with your urinary condition the way it is now, no better, no worse, for the rest of your life?	0	1	2	3	4	5	6

TOOLBOX

NOTES:

TOOLBOX

chapter THREE
Biopsy Results: What to Do?

"You can be a victim of cancer, or a survivor of cancer. It's a mindset.

— *Dave Pelzer, author and childhood abuse survivor*

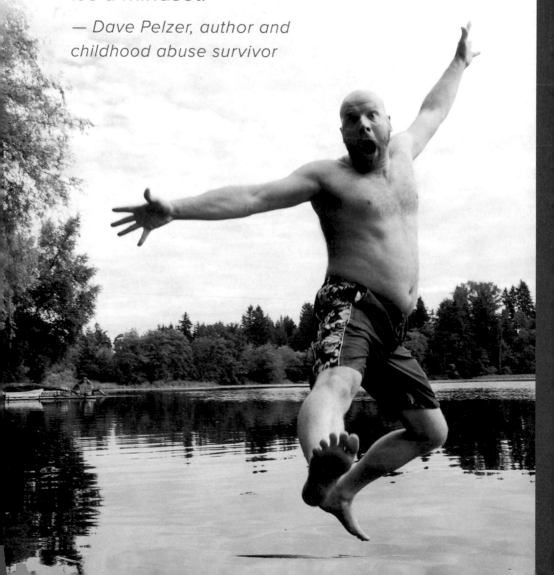

Patient Story

STEPHEN

What have I learned from my prostate cancer experience? Trust the science, but also trust your heart. Gather information, but listen to your intuition.

At 64, I was a healthy soon-to-be-retired public school administrator who was looking forward to becoming a full-time recreational cyclist. Prostate cancer was a shock.

For some reason, I thought I ought to have a physical. Nothing was wrong, it had just been a while. The blood work showed an elevated PSA, so my physician suggested the urologist downstairs, who'd likely order a prostate biopsy. Somewhere, I'd heard about too many unnecessary prostate biopsies; it was enough to make me hesitate.

My wife suggested another urologist, so I made an appointment. My new urologist thoroughly explained all the tests, and did recommend a prostate biopsy when the results of other tests suggested that this was the right step. The biopsy was positive for cancer.

You could say that I only delayed the process by not following my first doctor's advice ... but that would be missing the point.

I have always sought a balanced approach between science and the forces that science can't explain. The most important events of my life have taught me to pay attention to seemingly random events and decisions because of how easily they turn into "circumstances" of major significance.

If I reverse engineer my cancer experience, the most important parts are (1) an early diagnosis and (2) being referred for CyberKnife treatment. The science, the physics and the medicine did the trick. But I had to get there. I don't know if the urologist I chose NOT to see would have made that recommendation; however, I do know that all the other treatment options were invasive and had significant side effects. It had to be CyberKnife, so I could heal and go on with my life relatively unscathed.

chapter
THREE
summary

Chapter 3 helps you understand the information from a prostate biopsy. We also introduce you to the most common types of prostate cancer.

Our goal is to help you become a well-informed patient so you can ask the right questions and have better conversations with your doctor(s).

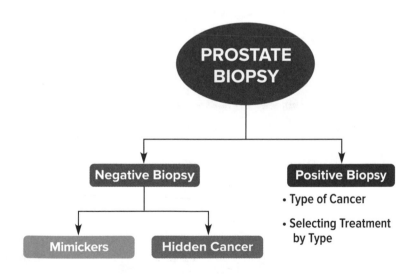

The third tier of **Figure 3.0** illustrates why a prostate cancer biopsy may not be a simple on/off, yes/no kind of procedure. Thanks to several new "epigenetic" and "genomic" tests, we can now separate prostate cancer from other conditions that have similar symptoms (mimickers), detect "hidden" prostate cancer (and detect it sooner) — and accurately determine how aggressive the cancer is once it's found.

DEBUNKING MYTHS

DOES A NEGATIVE PROSTATE BIOPSY MEAN YOU DO NOT HAVE PROSTATE CANCER? NOT ALWAYS ...

Of the 1.2 million prostate biopsies performed in the United States every year, over 700,000 (68%) are negative. Twenty-five percent of those 700,000 actually contain cancer.

Most of what a prostate biopsy tells you is whether the hollow-core needles that collected samples from your prostate DID or DID NOT detect any cancer.

Is it possible that these needles missed a tiny tumor of prostate cancer? Absolutely! Traditional prostate biopsies only sample 1% of the total prostate volume.

If you have any of the following, then there is good reason to repeat a negative prostate biopsy. Any of these results could indicate the presence of prostate cancer:

- *Elevated total PSA*
- *Low free PSA*
- *Rising PSA velocity*
- *Rising PSA density*
- *Higher 4KScore Test result*
- *Abnormal PCA3 or SelectMDx score*
- *Positive ConfirmMDx test*

The "false-negative" scenario mentioned above is exactly why 3D MRI fusion prostate biopsies are such a welcomed improvement over conventional random TRUS biopsies.

MRI fusion biopsies catch prostate cancer 70-75% of the time on the first biopsy, while conventional TRUS biopsies only catch cancer 30-35% of the time on the first biopsy.

Pairing an MRI picture of the prostate with a real-time ultrasound image also allows doctors to search suspicious areas and find hidden tumors that may have been missed on previous negative biopsies.

In addition, MRI fusion biopsies are 2-3 times more sensitive in detecting "clinically significant" prostate cancer and twice as accurate as standard TRUS biopsies in determining the extent of the cancer.

Combining MRI fusion technology with other tests like ConfirmMDx, SelectMDx, 4Kscore Test, and PCA3 gives doctors an increased chance of uncovering hidden and aggressive cancers.

VOCABULARY

See Glossary for Definitions

4Kscore Test	PIN (Prostatic Interstitial Neoplasia)
Bone Scan	PNI (Perineural Invasion)
ConfirmMDx	Prolaris
Decipher	Prostate Biopsy
DRE (Digital Rectal Exam)	PSA (Prostate Specific Antigen)
Epigenetic Testing	PSA Density
Extracapsular Extension (ECE)	PSA Free
False Negative	PSA Test
Genomic Testing	PSA Total
Gleason Score	PSA Velocity
Lymph Node	SelectMDx
Methylation	Seminal Vesicle Involvement
MRI	TRUS Prostate Biopsy
MRI Fusion Prostate Biopsy	Ultrasound
Oncotype DX	
PCA3 Test (urine)	

A NEW ERA IN PROSTATE CANCER DIAGNOSIS AND TREATMENT

Prostate cancer diagnosis and treatment are swiftly moving beyond Gleason Scores, PSA, Cancer Stages, and Partin Tables.

Today, blood biomarker tests like the 4Kscore Test, non-invasive urine-based molecular tests such as PCA3 and SelectMDx, epigenetic tests such as ConfirmMDx, image analysis tools like ProMark, and genomic tests such as OncotypeDX provide doctors with the tools to detect prostate cancer earlier and with greater accuracy than ever before.

These innovations allow patients to avoid unnecessary biopsies, while improving doctors ability to locate existing cancers. This improved accuracy helps doctors avoid overtreating insignificant cancers and undertreating cancers that have the potential to spread outside the prostate — even though these cancers initially appear to be low-risk.

As a patient, you want to know the true nature of your cancer, so you can find the best treatment for the kind of cancer you have.

Bottom line: We want all men who have "clinically significant" prostate cancer to get the best possible treatment. This is especially true for men with moderate- and high-risk disease. We also do NOT want to see men with "clinically insignificant" or "low-risk, low-volume" disease get over-treated and suffer life-altering complications from their treatment.

WHAT A BIOPSY LOOKS LIKE

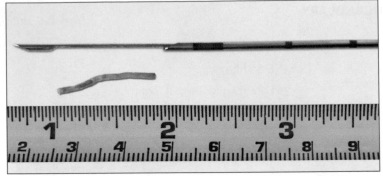

Figure 3.1 shows the actual shape and size of a prostate biopsy sample (often called a "needle core") and the biopsy needle itself. Normally, 12-24 of these samples are taken during a standard biopsy.

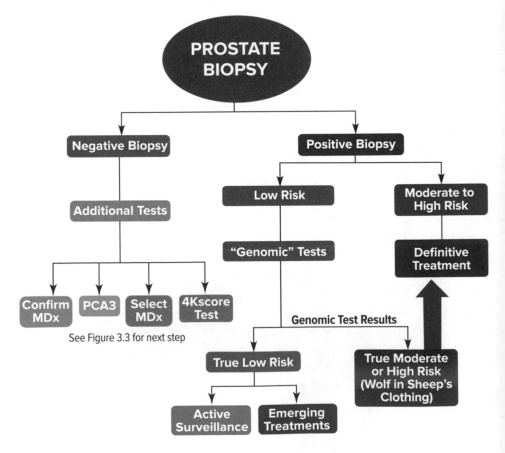

Figure 3.2 provides an overview of all the different tests and options based on whether your prostate biopsy comes back negative or positive.

BIOPSY RESULTS

WHAT TO DO WITH YOUR BIOPSY RESULTS

If your prostate biopsy is negative, one of three things is likely:

1. You do not have cancer

2. You have BPH and/or prostatitis.

3. The cancer is undetected

If your biopsy is positive, then it's time to make some choices about treatment options based on the kind of cancer you have. (We encourage you to look at the list of "12 Factors that Define Prostate Cancer" on **Page 75**).

The rest of this chapter is devoted to helping you understand how to interpret the results of your prostate biopsy.

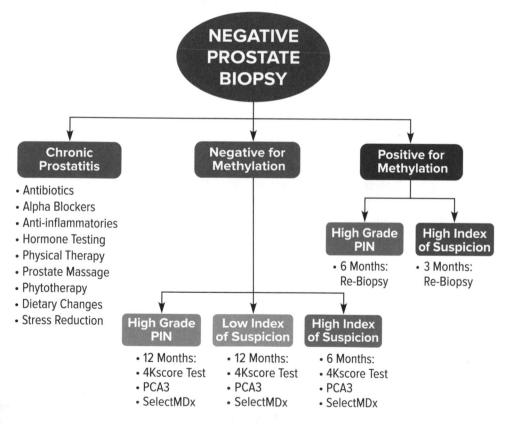

Figure 3.3 further explores the **possible scenarios** for a negative prostate biopsy and the additional next steps. **(This figure outlines some of your options. Not every test listed here is appropriate.)** "Index of Suspicion" means how likely you are to have cancer. For example, a low index of suspicion means a low probability of having prostate cancer, and a high index of suspicion means you have a high probability of having cancer. See **Page 72** for information on "Methylation."

NEGATIVE BIOPSY (NO CANCER)

> ### WHAT YOU NEED TO KNOW ABOUT METHYLATION
>
> *A new generation of "epigenetic" tests are able to evaluate prostate biopsy tissue samples for the presence or absence of "methylation." A positive methylation test suggests the presence of prostate cancer. A negative methylation test suggests the absence of prostate cancer.*

A negative biopsy means that your prostate biopsy showed no signs of cancer — which is great news!

Before you pop the champagne, however, we offer a few words of caution. Don't get us wrong, having a negative biopsy is a wonderful thing, it just does not completely rule out the presence of cancer.

If you've had a negative biopsy, we recommend that you talk with your doctor about where you fit in **Figure 3.3**:

1. No Cancer (most likely BPH or prostatitis)

2. Negative for methylation

3. Positive for methylation

This conversation with your doctor will be tempered by whether your doctor thinks you have a "low index of suspicion" (meaning you probably do NOT have prostate cancer — or if you do, it's a very low-grade cancer) or a "high index of suspicion," (meaning you probably DO have cancer, but it has not been detected yet.)

We see having a negative biopsy with a negative methylation test and a low index of suspicion as an opportunity to address your current lifestyle and learn how you can modify it to improve your health and prevent prostate cancer (See **Chapter 4**).

On the other hand, we see a negative biopsy with a positive methylation test and a high index of suspicion as a likely "false negative" biopsy (a biopsy that does not detect cancer, even though cancer is present).

A high index of suspicion usually prompts your doctor to recommend another round of tests (blood, urine, and DRE) and an additional prostate biopsy in 3-6 months.

Also, relatively new blood tests such as the 4Kscore Test, urine tests like Select MDx, and biopsy-based tests like ConfirMDx can help reveal the presence of hidden cancers that may be lurking in a "false negative" biopsy.

These innovative tests are so important is because traditional TRUS prostate biopsies only detect 30-35 percent of clinically significant prostate cancers on the first biopsy. MRI Fusion biopsies detect 70-75 percent of clinically significant prostate cancer on the first biopsy — which cuts down on the need for multiple biopsies (and the complications they create). However, MRI Fusion biopsies still miss 25-30 percent of cancers on the first try.

If you need to repeat a biopsy, we highly recommend that you ask your doctor if MRI fusion prostate biopsy technology is available in your area — or just Google "MRI fusion prostate biopsy" + your area or nearest city.

POSITIVE BIOPSY

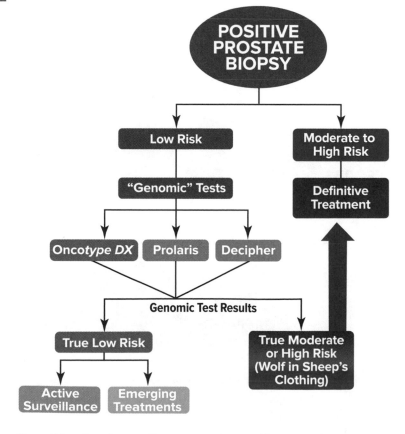

Figure 3.4 outlines the possible next steps after a positive prostate biopsy reveals low-risk, moderate-risk, or high-risk prostate cancer.

If any of the tissue samples taken during your prostate biopsy are positive for cancer, then you have some form of prostate cancer.

If that is the case, the next step is to answer these three questions:

1. **What type of cancer is it?**
2. **How much cancer was discovered?**
3. **What is the risk of this cancer developing into life-threatening (metastatic) disease?**

With the answers to these three questions, you're off to a good start toward selecting the right type of prostate cancer treatment for you and the kind of cancer you have. As you can see on the next page, additional information allows you to further refine your treatment options so you can select the best one for you.

Thanks to new genomic tests like Decipher, Onco*type* DX, and Prolaris, automated image recognition testing like ProMark, and urine/DRE tests like PCA-3 and Select MDx, doctors can now answer question #3 above with much greater certainty.

TYPES OF PROSTATE CANCER

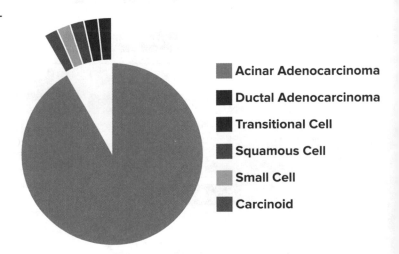

- Acinar Adenocarcinoma
- Ductal Adenocarcinoma
- Transitional Cell
- Squamous Cell
- Small Cell
- Carcinoid

Figure 3.5 Since the vast majority (95 percent) of prostate cancer is Acinar Adenocarcinoma, it's easy to lose sight of the fact that there are the five other types of prostate cancer, each of which requires its own treatment protocol.

> ## 95% OF PROSTATE CANCER IS ACINAR ADENOCARCINOMA
>
> *Throughout this book, when we talk about "prostate cancer," we are really talking about "Acinar Adenocarcinoma." Actually, there are 5 other kinds of prostate cancer (See* **Figure 3.5**). *Each of these cancers is unique, require its own treatment protocol, and represents about 1% of all prostate cancers.*

12 FACTORS THAT DEFINE PROSTATE CANCER

To answer the three questions on the previous page (and expand on them), pathologists, urologists, and other doctors look at the following 12 factors:

1. **Gleason Score:** How aggressive your cancer appears under a microscope
2. **PSA Total:** Your highest level
3. **Clinical Stage:** How your cancer was discovered
4. **Number of Positive Biopsy Samples**
5. **Highest Percent of Cancer Detected**
6. **Bilateral Positive Biopsy Samples** (Did your biopsy find positive samples come on both sides of the prostate? If "yes," how many from each side?)
7. **Location of Positive Biopsy Cores**
8. **Perineural Invasion** (Has the cancer invaded the nerves that travel through the prostate? Yes/No)
9. **Extracapsular Extension** (Does the cancer extend into or beyond the prostate membrane? Yes/No)
10. **Seminal Vesicle Involvement** (Yes/No)
11. **Positive Lymph Nodes** (Yes/No)
12. **Positive Bone Scan** (Yes/No)

By evaluating these 12 factors, doctors can categorize your cancer and give you a better explanation of:

- How much cancer is there
- Where the cancer is located
- What's the risk of it spreading outside your prostate
- Whether or not the cancer has already spread outside your prostate
- And a lot more

CANCER TYPE	LOW-RISK	MODERATE-RISK	HIGH-RISK
"CAT NAME"	KITTY CAT	BOBCAT	MOUNTAIN LION
Treatments	Observation or Single Treatment	Single or Dual Treatment	Dual Treatment + Hormones
Gleason Score	3+3 = 6	3+4 or 4+3 = 7	8-10
PSA	Less than 10	10-20	More than 20
Cancer Stage	T1 or T2A	T2B	T2C

Figure 3.6 shows the three traditional cancer markers (Gleason Score, PSA, and Cancer Stage) for clinically significant prostate cancer (low-risk, moderate-risk, and high-risk) and Dr. Ripoll's "Cat Names."

UNDERSTANDING CANCER THROUGH ANALOGIES

Over the years, Dr. Ripoll found that certain patients simply could not take in any more "medical information" after they received a prostate cancer diagnosis. So she gave the three main risk types of local prostate cancer (cancer that is still confined inside the prostate) "cat names." This way of talking about cancer was easier and more intuitive for some patients because it bypassed using a lot of numbers and medical terminology.

The "cat names" shown below are Dr. Ripoll's way of taking the emotional charge off a diagnosis and helping her patients find a little breathing room.

It's a lot harder to freak out about being labeled a "Kitty Cat" than it is to be told you have Gleason 3 + 3, T1C, PSA: 2.5, 5% in 1 of 18 core samples, low-risk, low-volume prostate cancer. The cat analogies cut through all the abbreviations, acronyms, and mumbo jumbo.

- Clinically Insignificant Prostate Cancer: **Kitten**
- Low-risk Prostate Cancer: **Kitty Cat**
- Moderate-risk Prostate Cancer: **Bobcat**
- High-risk Prostate Cancer: **Mountain Lion**

Dr. Ripoll's "cat names" are useful analogies for lots of men, but they don't work for everyone. If you don't like cats (or even if you do), we invite you to come up your own names for different kinds of cancer.

So far, we've heard "The pit bull to poodle spectrum"; "Papa bear, momma bear, baby bear"; and "Birds, rabbits, and turtles."

We invite you to you come up with your own names for different classifications of prostate cancer. Because your analogies might work perfectly for someone else, we would like to hear about the names you create.

Bottom line: Use whatever analogy helps you deal with your prostate cancer diagnosis.

NOTE

With or without analogies, receiving a prostate cancer diagnosis almost always feels overwhelming. We wrote **Chapter 9** *in* **Prostate Cancer: A New Approach to Diagnosis, Treatment, and Health** *specifically to help men and their families deal with the emotional upheaval of finding out you have cancer.*

If you have been diagnosed with prostate cancer, we highly recommend you purchase this more in-depth book or ask your doctor to provide you with a copy. It goes into much greater detail about the different kinds of prostate cancer, the latest types of prostate cancer treatment, and how to cope with your diagnosis.

Also, we encourage you to continue on to **Chapter 4** *in this book, because no matter what kind of prostate condition you have (prostatitis, BPH, cancer, or something else), the information in* **Chapter 4** *can help you heal your prostate — and your life.*

NEGATIVE BIOPSY

	What does it do?	How does it do it?
Confirm MDx	• Helps identify men who have prostate cancer that was undetected by a biopsy (false negative biopsy). False negative biopsies occur in about 25% of negative biopsies. • Points to specific areas of the prostate that are likely to contain cancer. • Decreases the number of unnecessary biopsies. • Used only with patients who have had negative biopsies.	• Detects areas within prostate biopsy samples that contain a higher concentration of "methylation." (A biochemical process that can shut down tumor-suppressors genes.) • Methylation may be present even though the prostate cells look normal under a microscope. • The confirmation of a methylation halo (also called a "field effect") points to the area(s) most likely to harbor hidden cancer.

Mentioned by name in **Figure 3.2** and indirectly in **Figure 3.3** (positive and negative for "methylation"), **Figure 3.7** provides a brief outline of what the Confirm MDx test does and how it works.

POSITIVE BIOPSY

The following three tests are examples of genomic tests. What is a genomic test? Good question. These tests are for men who have had a positive prostate biopsy. The tests measure the expression of certain DNA strands (called "genes") that are associated with aggressive prostate cancer — or the RNA strands that these genes create. For example, Onco*type* DX measures the expression of 17 such genes, Prolaris measures the expression of 46 genes, and Decipher measures 22 RNA biomarkers.

All three of these tests provide you with a score (a number) that explains how likely your prostate cancer is to grow rapidly and spread outside your prostate — where it is much harder to treat.

	What does it do?	How does it do it?
Oncotype DX	• A test for men who have recently been diagnosed with early-stage prostate cancer. • A medical breakthrough for men who had a positive prostate biopsy that found low-risk prostate cancer. Onco*type* DX uses the prostate biopsy sample to confirm that you have true low-risk prostate cancer – and not a more aggressive form of prostate cancer that is masquerading as low-risk cancer. • Gives patients a "Genomic Prostate Score" (GPS) that accurately predicts how aggressive a prostate cancer tumor is. • Adds valuable information that goes beyond Gleason Score and PSA.	• Onco*type* DX is a biopsy-based test that measures the level of expression of 17 aggressive prostate cancer genes. • It is performed on positive tissue samples from your most recent biopsy. The result is an individualized number called a "Genomic Prostate Score" (GPS). • Using these 17 prostate cancer genes, the GPS predicts how likely a man's prostate cancer is going to spread beyond his prostate. • This test can use tissue samples from a prostate biopsies or a radical prostatectomy (surgery).

POSITIVE BIOPSY continued

	What does it do?	How does it do it?
Prolaris	• As with Oncotype DX, Prolaris is a tissue-based molecular test that provides men with a way to determine how aggressive their prostate cancer is. Prolaris works in conjunction with traditional clinical prostate tests like Gleason Score and PSA. • Helps identify low- to moderate-risk patients. This information identifies good candidates for active surveillance versus candidates for definitive treatment. • This test can test both specimens from a prostate biopsy or a radical prostatectomy (surgery).	• It is a 46-gene test designed to gauge the aggressiveness of prostate cancer in individual patients. It measures the expression of genes that govern how quickly cells divide and make new cells. • Measures the expression of genes involved in cancer tumor proliferation to predict whether a man's cancer will eventually spread outside his prostate.
Decipher (after surgery)	• Analyzes a small tissue sample that is routinely taken during surgery and archived by the pathology laboratory. • Provides an independent assessment of tumor aggressiveness and predicts the probability of prostate cancer developing in other parts of the body after surgery (metastasis). • Provides Information independent from Gleason Score or PSA.	• Measures the expression of 22 RNA biomarkers involved in biological pathways that are associated with aggressive prostate cancer • Uses the expression of these biomarkers to calculate the probability of clinical metastasis within 5 years after surgery, and within 3 years of a rising PSA after surgery. • Has been validated by over 2,000 patients in clinical studies at top U.S. cancer centers.

Genomic Testing in a Nutshell

Some insurance companies cover one test but not the other two. Some doctors prefer one test over the others. If you have had a positive prostate biopsy, we recommend that you use whichever test your health insurance covers and your doctor recommends.

Figure 3.8 provides an outline of the three most common genomic tests: Onco*type* DX, Prolaris, and Decipher. These tests are given to men who have had a positive prostate biopsy to determine how aggressive their cancer is. Two of these tests, Onco*type* DX and Prolaris, can be used on positive prostate biopsy samples to identify aggressive prostate cancer that is masquerading as low-risk cancer. All three of these tests can be performed on prostate tissue samples after the prostate has been surgically removed. The results of all three tests can help men decide on the most appropriate next step in their treatment plan.

Doctor Story
DR. LEE MCNEELY, MD

Radiation Oncology
St Vincent Frontier
Cancer Center,
Billings, Montana

My patient, Jerry, is a healthy, physically active man in a vibrant relationship with his wife. The day he arrived for his initial radiation therapy consultation; however, he looked anything but his robust self.

We talked about prostate cancer specifics like Gleason score, PSA, tumor extent on biopsy — all indicating he had a very good prognosis for complete recovery.

As doctors, we naturally assume that this kind of news would be a welcomed relief. The look on Jerry's face, however, told a different story.

I noticed a change in Jerry as the conversation shifted to treatment options, which can be confusing with all the different types of radiation treatment available — seeds, external beam, combination protocols (both with and without hormonal therapy), and so on.

The more I talked about treatment options, the more relaxed Jerry became; it was as if someone had lifted a weight from his shoulders. "You mean I don't have to have surgery? Doc, I just don't want to be cut on 'down there.'"

Suddenly, he was a new man.

The more medicine advances, the more tools we have that empower patients to make healthy choices about their care and their lives. Some patients feel burdened by the responsibility making the "right choice." For those patients, know that doctors struggle with that challenge every day.

Today, Jerry is alive and well after his seed implantation (Brachytherapy). He recovered quickly from the irritating urinary symptoms. In follow-up visits, he thanked me every time for helping him make the right choice. And my reply was always the same, "You did that, Jerry. Not me."

LOOKING AHEAD

CHAPTER 1: You or your doctor is concerned about your prostate — We provide you with **Prostate 101**: where it lives, what it does, plus relevant statistics.

CHAPTER 2: Your doctor told you to **schedule a prostate biopsy** — We give you a **Prostate Biopsy Assessment Tool** to see if you actually need one, and what to expect if you do.

CHAPTER 3: You have a prostate biopsy — We explain the steps you need to take, whether you have a **negative biopsy or a positive biopsy**.

CHAPTER 4: You want to **use your cancer diagnosis as a springboard to better health** — We help you address your wellness goals with a proven plan that covers inflammation, diet, inactivity, stress, immune system, hormones, structure, and removing toxic substances.

WHAT'S NEXT?

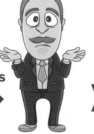

I Need Help with My Overall Health & Wellness
Go To Chapter 4

I Had a Positive Biopsy
Get a Second Opinion

I Need More Information
Read *Prostate Cancer: A New Approach...*

WELCOME TO THE TOOLBOX
CHAPTER 3 **TOOLBOX**

THIS TOOLBOX SECTION INCLUDES THE FOLLOWING TOOLS AND RESOURCES TO HELP YOU UNDERSTAND THE RESULTS OF YOUR PROSTATE BIOPSY:

- Call List of Important People
- Prostate Cancer Resources List

Call List

	NAME	NUMBER
FAMILY		
FRIENDS		
COUNSELOR/ THERAPIST		
RELIGIOUS ADVISOR		
PRIMARY DOCTOR		
UROLOGIST		
SECOND OPINION		
THIRD OPINION		
NUTRITIONIST		
SUPPORT GROUP		
INSURANCE BENEFITS		
WORK BENEFITS		
FINANCIAL ADVISOR		

TOOLBOX

Prostate Cancer Resources

We include this alphabetical list as a resource for additional information. Unfortunately, we cannot guarantee that any of these resources will be helpful in your search for leading-edge information about prostate health, prostate cancer, its treatment, or a community to support you in your search; however, we have generally found these resources to be helpful.

CANCER TREATMENT CENTERS OF AMERICA
http://www.cancercenter.com/prostate-cancer

CANCER COMPASS PROSTATE CANCER DISCUSSIONS
www.cancercompass.com/message-board/cancers/prostate-cancer/1,0,119,2.htm

CANCER HOPE NETWORK   1-877-467-3638
www.cancerhopenetwork.org
Matches cancer patients one-on-one with someone who has recovered from a similar experience.

DAILY STRENGTH PROSTATE CANCER SUPPORT GROUP
www.dailystrength.org/c/Prostate-Cancer/support-group

IMERMAN ANGELS   1-877-274-5529
www.imermanangels.org
Imerman Angels partners a person fighting cancer with someone who has beaten the same type of cancer.

MALE CARE
www.malecare.org

MALECARE: MODERATED EMAIL DISCUSSION LISTS
health.groups.yahoo.com/group/prostatecancerunder50
health.groups.yahoo.com/group/prostatecancerandgaymen
health.groups.yahoo.com/group/advancedprostatecancer

NATIONAL CANCER INSTITUTE LIFELINE
http://www.cancer.gov/cancertopics/disparities/lifelines/prostatecancer

OUT WITH CANCER: ONLINE LGBT COMMUNITY
http://www.outwithcancer.org

PROSTATE CANCER FOUNDATION
http://www.pcf.org

TOOLBOX

PROSTATE CANCER FOUNDATION — SUPPORT GROUPS
http://www.pcf.org/site/c.leJRIROrEpH/b.5856543/k.6599/Finding_a_Support_Group.htm

PROSTATE CANCER RESEARCH INSTITUTE
http://www.pcri.org

PROSTATE CANCER: VOLUME, DIMENSION & DENSITY
http://www.mskcc.org/nomograms/prostate/volume

PROSTATE CONDITIONS EDUCATION COUNCIL
https://prostateconditions.org

PROSTATE HEALTH EDUCATION NETWORK
http://www.prostatehealthed.org

PSA DOUBLING TIME
http://www.mskcc.org/nomograms/prostate/psa-doubling-time

THE SCOTT HAMILTON CARES INITIATIVE   1-866-520-3197
4TH ANGEL PROGRAM
http://www.4thangel.org

Free, national service that provides a one-to-one supportive relationship (phone or email) to cancer patients and their caregivers.

US TOO PROSTATE CANCER SUPPORT GROUP
http://www.ustoo.org

US TOO INSPIRE ONLINE COMMUNITY
www.inspire.com/inspire/group/us-too-prostate-cancer

YANA - YOU ARE NOT ALONE
NOW PROSTATE CANCER SUPPORT SITE
www.yananow.org

ZERO: THE END OF PROSTATE CANCER
https://zerocancer.org

TOOLBOX

chapter **FOUR**

Using Your Diagnosis as a Springboard to Better Health

To find health should be the object of the doctor. Anyone can find disease.

Dr. Andrew Taylor Still, MD
Father of Osteopathic Medicine

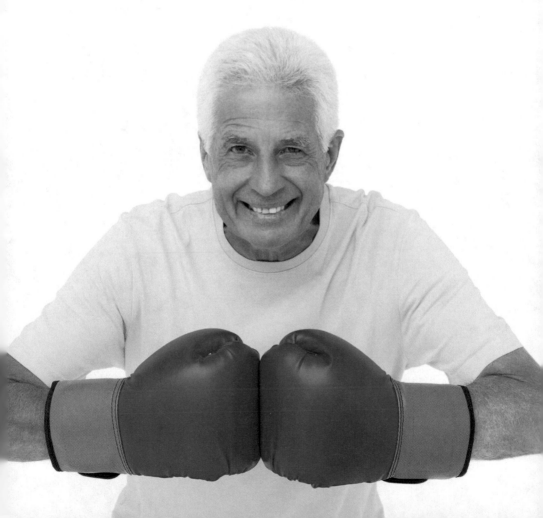

Patient Story

JEFF

I am one of the fortunate people who have overcome prostate cancer and now live a cancer-free life. While cancer is not a journey that I would wish on anyone, I do feel that it has taught me 10 profound lessons.

1. The diagnosis can be overwhelming

It doesn't matter what type, what stage, or at what age, getting cancer is no fun. One day you're feeling fine, life is normal, and the next day your doctor tells you that you have cancer. And that's just the beginning: Doctor visits, expensive tests, treatment options, big decisions, and a wicked learning curve in "doctor speak" — and that's just the physical side. Cancer is also mentally, emotionally, and spiritually draining.

2. Some things are beyond our control

Cancer affects people from all walks of life. You can minimize the risk of cancer, but you can't control what life throws your way. You can, however, control how you deal with those curve balls.

3. It's a wake-up call

If being told you have a disease that could kill you doesn't make you take stock of your life, then I don't know what will. Cancer made me realize that life is precious and not to be taken for granted. It made me think about my purpose on this planet, the life I want to live, the people I want to touch, and the legacy I want to leave.

4. Cancer doesn't define me

Yes, I am a cancer survivor, but that label doesn't define me. I am more than a disease. I was a vibrant person before being diagnosed, and am even more so now.

5. Cancer is a gift

It might sound cliché, but I see my cancer as a gift. It has brought me closer to my kids and deepened my relationship with my wife. I have received love and compassion from unexpected people and in unexpected ways. It has opened me up to feeling more empathy for others.

6. Cancer knows no boundaries
Cancer can affect anyone at any time; I know athletes in peak physical shape, children, grandparents, and people from all walks of life who have been diagnosed.

When I was diagnosed, I was in great shape, ate a healthy diet, exercised regularly, and did not have a single symptom. My dad had prostate cancer, so I knew that I had a higher chance of getting it.

7. Appreciate the little things in life
Not long after my diagnosis, I remember pulling off to the side of the road to watch a flock of birds overhead. I remember stopping in the middle of a bike ride to pet and feed a horse. It wasn't until after I had cancer that I really started to take notice of the finer things in life, things that I was either too busy to notice or took for granted.

8. Life is short
Cancer woke me up to how short a run we have on this planet. Prior to cancer, I hadn't thought about my mortality. Cancer changed that. I realize that I had an end date, and no matter which life I wanted to create, the time to act was now.

9. It raised my level of empathy
Surviving cancer made me a more empathetic person. I am a lot less judgmental after I realized that I have no idea what path other people are on, or what they have to endure every day.

10. I am not alone
According to the American Cancer Society, the lifetime risk of developing cancer for men in the United States is slightly less than 1 in 2, for women a little more than 1 in 3. These numbers tell us how close to home cancer actually is, and they have prompted an unprecedented level of research, care, treatment, and understanding of this disease.

Unknowingly, my cancer journey has been a path of personal growth. It has had a huge impact on my quality of life and my ability to appreciate how blessed my life truly is.

VOCABULARY

See Glossary for Definitions

Bladder

Bio-individuality

BPH (Benign Prostatic Hyperplasia)

Brainspotting

Cortisol (pro-inflammatory hormone)

Digital Rectum Exam (DRE)

DHEA (Dehydroepiandroste-rone)

DHT (Dihydro-testosterone)

DNA (Deoxyribonucleic acid)

EMDR (Eye Movement Desen-sitization and Reprocessing)

Emotional Freedom Technique Hormones

Functional Medicine Doctor

Gene

Gleason Score

GMO: Genetically Modified Organisms

Insulin

Muscle Activation Technique

Mutation

Neuromodulation Technique

Pelvic Floor

PIN (Prostatic Intraepithelial Neoplasia)

Prostate Biopsy

Prostate Cancer

Prostate Zones

PSA (Prostate Specific Antigen)

PSA Testing

Rectum

Seminal Vesicles

Seminal Vesicle Fluid

Standard American Diet

Trans Fat

Urethra

Urinary Retention

Urinary Sphincter

Western Diet

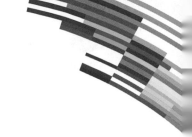

chapter
FOUR
summary

We included **Chapter 4** because we know how important it is to have everyday tools that help you address your prostate problems.

Whether you have received a prostate cancer diagnosis or had your negative prostate biopsy validated by tests like ConfirmMDx, the 7 point plan in **Chapter 4** acts like a springboard to better health — better prostate health and better overall health.

We highly recommend that you use the information in this chapter to jump-start your journey back to health.

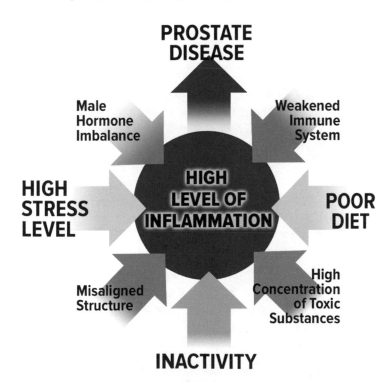

Figure 4.0 is an easy way to visualize how interconnected the seven health factors mentioned in this chapter are. They can either work together to promote prostate cancer by increasing inflammation (as in this figure) or to reduce inflammation and promote prostate health (as in **Figure 4.2**).

7 FACTORS THAT DECREASE INFLAMMATION AND REDUCE THE RISK OF PROSTATE CANCER

1. Diet   2. Inactivity   3. Stress   4. Structure
5. Immune System   6. Hormones   7. Toxic Substances

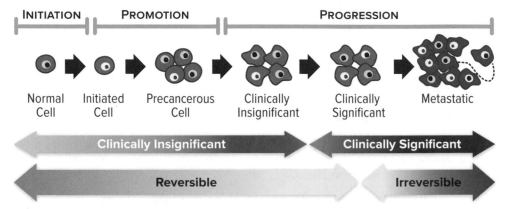

Figure Intro 1.1 visually displays how plastic the process of developing prostate cancer is.
Bottom line: Prostate cancer is treatable, and in some cases reversible, if caught early enough.

DEBUNKING MYTHS

PROSTATE CANCER IS IRREVERSIBLE

*Perhaps the most important information in **Figure Intro 1.1** (above), is that prostate cancer is **REVERSIBLE**, especially in its early stages.*

Thankfully, new scientific research about active surveillance and its affect on prostate cancer has demonstrated that an anti-cancer lifestyle can actually reverse prostate cancer. It all depends upon where a man is on the spectrum of disease (see figure above), plus his age, general health, and a few other factors.

For many people, including some doctors, the idea that prostate cancer is reversible remains controversial.

The location of the line between reversible and irreversible prostate cancer varies from man to man. In general, we consider low-risk, low-volume prostate cancer to be reversible with active surveillance. Other risk factors such as the patient's age, overall health, pelvic health, and any previous pelvic surgeries are also part of the equation.

Also, it's important to realize that there's a big difference between "reversible" and "treatable." Prostate cancer that is not "reversible" may be very "treatable," with a high treatment success rate and minimal complications.

INFLAMMATION

	Problems	Solutions
Inflammation	1. Immune System	1. Treat infections & prostatitis
	2. Diet	2. Eat a low-glycemic (low-sugar) diet
	3. Toxic Substances	3. See **Page 110**
	4. Inactivity	4. Exercise 30 minutes a day
	5. Structure	5. See **Page 108**
	6. Stress	6. Start a stress reduction program
	7. Hormones	7. Have your hormone levels and ratios checked by a certified functional medicine doctor
	8. Prostate	8. Begin our 7-point program

Figure 4.1 outlines the causes and solutions for inflammation — which is the root cause of many kinds of prostate disease — including cancer.

INFLAMMATION IS THE ORIGIN OF CHRONIC DISEASE.

Regaining your health after any kind of prostate disease diagnosis is all about reducing Inflammation and reversing its negative effects your body. This is no simple task.

Why? *Because inflammation occurs on every level of your body: whole body, organ systems, organs, cellular — even your DNA*. Diseases like obesity, heart disease, stroke, diabetes, and prostate cancer are all manifestations of inflammation.

The causes of inflammation are everywhere. The sources include the food we eat (high-glycemic diet), the stagnant way we work (sitting for hours), the stress we carry around (increased cortisol), our misaligned bodies, and our over-worked immune systems ... to the toxic chemicals we are subjected to in the food we eat, the water we drink, and the air we breathe.

The point of this chapter is to make you aware of how a poor diet, inactivity, high stress, malfunctioning immune system, out-of-balance hormone levels, postural problems, and the presence of toxic substances in your body all work together to create prostate disease (cancer).

Once you are aware of what the problems are, then you can take advantage of our seven-point plan to fix them, which is what the **Chapter 4 Toolbox** is all about.

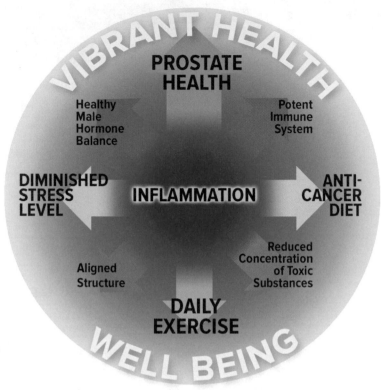

Figure 4.2 illustrates how the seven interconnected health areas mentioned in this chapter can work together to reduce inflammation and restore your overall health, as well as the health of your prostate.

If you want to regain your health, you're going to have to make some changes — and change is scary. It runs counter to our desire for comfort and what's familiar.

To help you take make the right changes, we offer you our seven-point plan to rid your body of inflammation and help heal your prostate.

Figure 4.2 (above) reverses the direction of the seven health factors listed in **Figure 4.0** (from promoting prostate cancer to reviving prostate health). These two figures point out how these seven interconnected areas can either be your enemies (**Figure 4.0**) or your friends (**Figure 4.2**).

Even if you have been undermining your health for decades, **Chapter 4** will give you the tools you need to rejuvenate and revitalize your life. It's all about awareness.

DIET

	Problems	Solutions
DIET	1. Insulin/sugar problems & toxic chemicals in food	1. Eat mostly organic vegetables (especially cruciferous vegetables) and low-glycemic fruit
	2. High-glycemic diet	2. Low-glycemic diet
	3. Growth hormone/antibiotics in food	3. Eat animal protein that is free of all hormones and antibiotics
	4. Processed foods and trans fats	4. Restore the balance between omega 3 & omega 6 fatty acids
	5. Grains	5. Limit grains and breads
	6. Poor quality oils	6. Use more olive and coconut oil
	7. Alcohol, sweetened sodas, and caffeine consumption	7. Limit alcohol, sodas, and caffeine

Figure 4.3 identifies a few of the many pitfalls that eating a "Western Diet" (Standard American Diet). Eating this way has a huge impact on inflammation and chronic diseases like diabetes, heart disease, strokes ... and prostate cancer.

Your diet is *the* easiest, fastest, and most powerful tool you have to improve your health. It is also the one thing you have complete control over. Unless you live in prison or are on a forced meal plan, you have complete control over what goes into your mouth.

Worldwide, the "Western Diet" is the single biggest cause of chronic disease. It is a recipe for inflammation with all of its processed foods, sweeteners and simple carbs, artificially modified oils, and meat that is awash in antibiotics and growth hormones.

To learn more about how your diet (and the other six health factors mentioned in this chapter) interact with your body, we encourage you to go to the **Chapter 4 Toolbox** and explore the interactive information there.

WHAT YOU DON'T EAT IS MORE IMPORTANT THAN WHAT YOU DO. AVOID THESE 5 FOODS TO REDUCE YOUR LEVEL OF INFLAMMATION:

1. Get Rid of Sweeteners

Sugar is a toxin. Why would you want to eat a toxin? (Because it tastes so sweet, obviously.)

Sugar and its metabolic equivalents (sweeteners) come in many forms: agave syrup, brown sugar, brown rice syrup, cane juice, fruit juice concentrate, high fructose corn syrup, honey, maple syrup, molasses, sucanat, turbinado … the list goes on.

Look at the food labels and see how many of these sweeteners are in your favorite foods. Sweeteners (except stevia) flood your body with sugar, which boosts the production of the hormone insulin. Insulin moves glucose out of your blood and into your tissues, instructs your body to store fat, and increases inflammation.

If you want to lose weight, heal from cancer (and several other diseases), maintain your mental edge, and generally feel healthy, *cut out sweeteners.* As painful as this advice may be, it's that simple.

2. Avoid Simple Carbs

Breads, pastas, breakfast cereals, granola, waffles, pancakes, cookies, crackers, popcorn, snack foods, candy, "energy' bars … even white potatoes are metabolized by your body the same way sugar is. They all boost insulin production, instruct your body to store fat, and promote inflammation at every level.

3. Say "Goodbye" to Grains

Grains generally cause the same sugar rush, insulin spike, fat storage, and inflammation as simple carbs.

This response is true for "whole grains" and gluten-free grains. If you're going to eat grains, however, go with gluten-free whole grains. They are easier to digest and contain more nutrients.

4. Don't Eat Dairy

Consider this: Humans are the only animals that continue to drink milk after we have been weaned from our mothers. We are also the only animals to regularly drink the milk of another animal (cows and goats, mostly).

Several European studies have show that men who eat 2-3 servings of dairy products per day are up to eight times more likely to develop prostate cancer.

5. Just Say "No" to Alcohol

Sugar is a toxin. Alcohol is a poison. Why would you want to poison your body when you're trying to heal from prostate cancer? That makes no sense.

In 1988, the World Health Organization classified alcohol as a Group 1 carcinogen. Regular heavy alcohol consumption increases the risk for seven different types of cancer, including prostate, breast, colorectal, oral, and liver.

NOTE

Before you begin any new diet, it's a good idea to get tested to see if you are allergic to certain foods. Food allergies/sensitivities create inflammation, so food allergy testing is a good place to start.

HERE ARE THE BIG 3 FOODS YOU SHOULD EAT TO REPLACE THE OTHER 5 YOU JUST CUT OUT OF YOUR DIET.

1. Eat Lots of Organic Vegetables and some Low-Glycemic Fruits

Your goal is to make your diet 60-75 percent organic, non-starchy vegetables and low-glycemic fruits. Think of 60-75 percent as five helpings (cups) of fresh vegetables and fruit per day (4 cups of vegetables and 1 of fruit). Your body will thank you for the rest of your life.

Include lots of cruciferous vegetables: broccoli, cauliflower, Brussels sprouts, bok choy, kale, cabbage ... and many others. These vegetables contain compounds that actually kill cancer.

Onions and garlic not only improve the taste of food, they have cancer-fighting properties as well.

Warning: The pesticides, herbicides, and fungicides in conventionally grown fruits and vegetables are poisons. No amount of rinsing will wash these poisons off — they are embedded in the body of the plant.

Warning: The results of feeding GMO (Genetically Modified Organism) food to lab animals are frightening. Avoid them wherever possible. Ask your grocer if your vegetables and fruit contain GMOs. If they don't know, don't buy it.

2. Healthy Fats Are Your Friends

A diet rich in animal fats and trans fats is one of the clearest dietary links to prostate cancer. These unhealthy fats clog the tiny arteries throughout your body and promote heart attacks, strokes, and erectile dysfunction. However, the healthy fats found in **avocados, seeds, and nuts** are important for hormone production, memory, smooth skin, and supple hair.

Healthy Fats: Olive oil, coconut oil, and clarified butter.

Unhealthy Fats: Margarine, trans-fats, cotton seed oil, soy oil, and safflower oil.

So-So Fats: Sesame oil, canola oil, and peanut oil.

3. **Clean, Lean Animal Protein Cooked at Low Temperatures is OK**

Several new studies show a connection between eating meat and developing cancer — specifically red meat, processed meat, and prostate cancer. Here's the information we think men concerned about prostate cancer need to know:

- If you eat animal protein, eat grass-fed, organic meat (or wild game/fish). The antibiotics, nitrates, and hormones in conventionally raised meats are linked to the rise of "super bugs," heart disease, and cancer.

- Avoid meat cooked at high temperatures (pan-seared, grilled, charred, deep fried, or blackened). Cooking at high temperatures creates compounds in the meat that promote prostate cancer.

- Cooking meat at high temperatures also makes the proteins and fats more difficult to digest.

- Avoid processed meats, luncheon meats, smoked meats, jerky, pastrami, bacon ... basically any meat that has been treated with anything. They are extremely unhealthy for your heart and your prostate.

- All the problems associated with eating meat multiply when you eat a lot of it. Instead of feasting on 1/2lb. burgers or 16 oz. steaks, eat smaller portions of meat (no bigger than a cigarette package).

- Eat the leanest meats you can find. Animal fat is a sponge for toxic substances and carcinogens.

- Several studies connect eating red meat with prostate cancer. However, we are unaware of any studies showing the negative effects of eating slow-cooked, grass-fed, organic red meat. More research on eating this kind of red meat would be valuable.

INACTIVITY

INACTIVITY	Problems	Solutions
	1. Chronic inflammation, pain, and habitual stress	1-3. Move your body: Stand up every hour, walk around, do chores, stay active
	2. Accumulation of toxic substances in excess body fat leads to being both overweight and unhealthy	1-3. Build your strength, endurance, and flexibility slowly over time. Exercise daily but avoid overtraining.
	3. Lack of exercise leads to stagnant circulation, fatigue, depression, and a diminished desire to move your body	1-3. Combine slow/steady exercise with resistance training and interval training, which improves circulation and removes toxic substances

Figure 4.4 points to why exercise is essential for a healthy body (and prostate), and inactivity is an evil habit that ruins your health and robs you of your energy.

EXERCISE IS A FEAST THAT NOURISHES THE BODY, ENLIVENS THE MIND, AND FREES THE SPIRIT.

We discuss the heart-prostate connection in *Prostate Cancer: A New Guide to Diagnosis, Treatment, and Health,* but for now, know that if something is good for your heart, it's probably good for your prostate, too.

The human body was designed to walk from place to place to gather food, sprint full speed when chasing after prey animals (or being chased by predators), and doing short bursts of all-out exercise (tree climbing, rock climbing, and fighting) followed by rest.

The value of this variety of daily exercise is most visible in its absence. In our increasingly sedentary culture many of us sit for 8-10 hours a day. The absence of daily physical activity is especially alarming considering that almost 70 percent people in the United States are overweight.

So, how do you incorporate exercise into your daily life?

NOTE

First and foremost: Always consult with your primary care physician, a physical therapist, or knowledgeable personal trainer before you embark on a new exercise regime. Talk with people who have a thorough understanding of any limitations you have, as well as proper exercise technique and the use of exercise equipment.

It's important to realize that there is no single kind of exercise that is best for everyone. To get the most out of the time you spend exercising, it's about integrating different kinds of exercise to train smarter — not harder.

Also keep in mind that you have to play the ball where it lies. **If walking around the block is all your body can handle at first, that's fine.** Persistence is the key. The longer you stay with a comprehensive exercise program, the more you will be able to increase your endurance, vitality, and cardiovascular health.

WE RECOMMEND A FOUR-PRONGED APPROACH:

1. **Breathe hard for at least 30 minutes every day.**
   Do something every day that makes you breathe so hard that it is difficult to hold a conversation. You may have to get up a half an hour earlier or skip some other activity that is NOT helping you improve your health. Don't stop if you miss a day. Daily exercise is the goal, but 3-4 times per week is a huge improvement over sitting on the sofa seven days a week.

2. **Resistance training is key to rebuilding your health.**
   When it comes to reducing inflammation, the value of pushing, pulling, lifting, and releasing some sort of resistance cannot be overemphasized.

   It doesn't matter if you are using your body weight or some kind of equipment that provides resistance (a weight machine or free weights). Stressing your core muscles (the ones responsible for alignment and posture) and your skeletal muscles (the ones that move your body) helps you build strength, muscular endurance, balance, maintain healthy hormone levels, get a good night's sleep, and generally feel better about life.

   Group classes help take the drudgery out of resistance training. Try Pilates, TRX, kettle balls, or any number of group fitness classes that use resistance.

   If classes don't work for you, then start a resistance training program by doing push-ups and core strength exercises on the floor during TV commercials.

Weight lifting (using weight machines or free weights) is an exceptional way to boost strength, tone your body, improve circulation, and reduce inflammation, all of which can have a positive impact on your prostate.

The way you workout is also important. Without going into the science of training, as a man with prostate problems, your goal is to maximize the health benefits of your workouts without pushing your body to the point where you either hurt yourself or you are too sore to exercise the following day.

No medals given for bravery: If you're hurt, you can't exercise. If you're too sore, you don't want to.

Rome was not built in a day. Neither was your temple. It's normal to jump into a new exercise program, especially after a health scare. The importance of a solid foundation cannot be overestimated. Go slow. Don't overdo it. Remember: The goal here is "healing."

3. High-intensity exercise achieves the same results in a fraction of the time.

What is high-intensity exercise? Think of it as short bursts of going as fast as you can without hurting yourself. For some people that's a 50 percent effort; for others, it's closer to 100 percent. This "flat out for 30 seconds" kind of exercise mimics what our ancestors did while hunting or avoiding being hunted.

We recommend 30 seconds of high-intensity exercise followed by 90 seconds to recover your breath and bring your heart rate back down. (You won't recover completely, but your breathing and heart rate will come back down.) Eight of these cycles (30 seconds of "all out" effort followed by 90 seconds of "active recovery") is ideal. In 16 minutes, you will achieve similar results from jogging for two hours.

You will probably have to build up to eight cycles. One cycle may be all you can do the first time — no problem. Simply add a cycle as you can until you're up to eight.

If it's been a while since you exercised or if you are obese, 30 seconds of high-intensity exercise might be just walking at a brisk pace, and your 90 seconds would be slowing it down to a stroll. If you're already in good shape, you could do this 30/90 seconds pattern while walking, running, swimming, cycling, hiking, on a rowing machine or an elliptical trainer.

This kind of interval training, does wonders for your heart, boosts your male hormone production, and improves your overall health.

Be careful: We recommend you start with one high-intensity session per week and build slowly to a maximum of three. Interval training can do wonders for your body (and mind). If done incorrectly, however, it's also an easy way to injure yourself.

Substitute one 16-minute high-intensity workout for one "breathe hard every day for 30-minutes" workout. This way, you vary your exercise patterns, which takes the drudgery out of working out.

4. **Keep Your Spine Supple (also see "STRUCTURE" later in this chapter)**

Healthy Pelvis — Happy Prostate

If your lower spine and pelvis are in good alignment and free from chronic pain, chances are the muscles and connective tissue in your pelvic floor will be strong yet supple. This kind of supple lower spine and pelvis allows for healthy blood and lymph circulation in and around the prostate gland, which promotes health and reduces inflammation.

There are several ways to improve how supple your lower back and pelvis are:

EXERCISES

- **Core strengthening**: Postural muscles
- **Flexibility training:** Yoga and stretching
- **Pilates & Gyrotonics:** Strengthens and elongates the spine through its full range of motion

HANDS-ON THERAPIES

- Physical Therapy
- Osteopathic/Chiropractic manipulation
- Acupuncture
- Rolfing
- Muscle Activation Technique
- Neurokinetic Therapy
- Craniosacral Therapy

If you are unfamiliar with these exercises or hands-on therapies, we recommend a simple Google search for which ones are available in your area.

NOTE

The biggest challenge with any new exercise program is avoiding injuries. That's why it is important to intentionally underachieve for the first couple of months.

As a man with prostate problems, it is far better to regain your health and fitness at a slightly slower pace than it is to get injured and not be able to receive the daily benefits of exercise and being active.

Yoga, hiking, swimming, weight lifting, Pilates, riding your bike ... are all wonderful activities that feel great and help your body heal. Just remember to take it easy for a while — there's no finish line here.

STRESS

	Problems	Solutions
STRESS	1. A prostate cancer diagnosis	1. The "right fit" prostate cancer treatment plan
	2. Fears about money and your close relationships	2. Seek sound financial advice and open up to the people closest to you
	3. Work-related issues	3. Talk with co-workers and supervisors (if you can)
	4. Feeling overwhelmed	4. Daily deep breathing practice promotes feeling calm
	5. Too much cortisol and adrenaline in your system	5. Daily exercise, limit stimulants, prayer/meditation

Figure 4.5 outlines common causes and solutions for chronic stress. Whatever your stress level was before a medical diagnosis, expect it to go up — especially if the diagnosis is prostate cancer. The trick is to learn new ways to cope with stress (the old stress & the new) so you can move forward on your healing path.

Stress comes in many forms:

- Health problems (like a prostate cancer diagnosis)
- Money issues
- Grief/Death of a loved one
- Losing a job
- Difficult relationships
- Challenges at work
- Taking care of aging parents or a high-needs child
- Getting married
- Getting divorced
- Living in uncertainty or fear
- Traumatic events (and the PTSD that follows)
- ... the list goes on

The connection between stress and cancer is well documented. It is our observation that many people who "get" cancer often go through an especially stressful period a year or two before they are diagnosed.

The net effect of chronic stress is that it stretches the body's immune system beyond its ability maintain your well being. In the absence of a robust immune system, the unhealthy processes going on inside our bodies gain the upper hand, and that's when we get sick.

Any kind of cancer diagnosis multiplies the level of stress you were experiencing before the diagnosis, which only makes matters worse.

Think of it this way, if your stress level contributed to developing cancer — then the additional stress of being diagnosed with cancer just sent your previous stress level into the stratosphere.

It is difficult to tease apart one source of stress from another because many of them involve other people or situations beyond your control. Instead of trying to bend the river, we recommend that you use these eight strategies to move with the current — not against it.

EIGHT PROVEN STRATEGIES FOR COPING WITH STRESS:

1. **Daily Exercise:** It's cheap, easy, and unless it is too painful to move your body for 30 minutes every day, every aspect of your life will benefit from exercise — especially your stress level.

2. **Connect with the People Who Love You:** You cannot put a price tag on the support you receive from the people (and animals) who love you. Surround yourself with these people and let them care for you in their own way. The support of spouses, partners, family, friends, pets, and your community helps create an environment where healing is possible.

3. **Eat Good Food:** Your body thrives on good nutrition. The simple act of nourishing your body cuts down on the insulin level in your body. Find a way to work cruciferous vegetables, fish and lean chicken, organic fruit, and healthy fats into your comfort foods.

   For example, oven-roasted Brussels sprouts, cauliflower, broccoli, a few cloves of garlic, with a dash of olive oil and balsamic vinegar on top is an easy and healthy meal (add a little pulled chicken or a can of tuna and you have a complete meal). Likewise, replace your nightly bowl of ice cream with the same bowl of organic fruit and berries with a handful of chopped almonds on top. Delicious!

4. **Prayer/Meditation:** If you are a prayerful person, then now would be the time to pray. If you're not, you can achieve a similar level of peace simply by sitting in a chair with your eyes closed while gently noticing the rise and fall of your breath. Two 20-minute sessions of prayer or meditation each day, can significantly shift your stress level and completely turn your life around. If one 20-minute session is all you can fit in, then that's a great place to start!

5. **Chi (Qi) Gong:** This ancient Chinese martial art combines the joy of exercise with the calm of meditation. Chi Gong uses breathing techniques, physical postures, precise motions, and focused intention (meditation) to help move the universal life energy (Chi) throughout your body.

   Chi Gong practice (which looks like its more well known cousin: Tai Chi) is part moving meditation and part slow-flowing movement accompanied by rhythmic breathing and a deeply relaxed state of mind.

6. The Smile

This technique comes from Chi Gong and is perfect for people who don't have a lot of time to devote to prayer or meditation. All that's required is a quiet place and five minutes.

All you have to do is close you eyes and think of something that makes you truly happy. This is not "fake it until you make it." You need to feel your body, especially the muscles of your face, smile. Then, you send that smile to your prostate and pelvis.

The best time to practice "The Smile" is when you wake up or when you go to sleep.

7. Therapeutic Techniques

The following techniques deliver outstanding results with people who are experiencing debilitating stress or Post Traumatic Stress Disorder (PTSD).

A prostate cancer diagnosis can create what feels like never-ending waves of stress or bring old traumas and painful memories to the surface so they can be healed.

Although healing old issues and past traumas is generally a good idea, sometimes the level of stress that comes up can feel overwhelming. That's when turning to a professional counselors trained in these techniques can be invaluable.

- **EMDR** (Eye Movement Desensitization and Reprocessing)
- **Brainspotting**
- **Emotional Freedom Technique**
- **Neuromodulation Technique**

The results of these therapies border on the miraculous, including reports of people healing from decades of stress and PTSD in as few as 5-10 sessions.

Patients frequently report that years of nagging thoughts and the endless replaying of painful images simply stop.

Patients often describe this sudden shift, like they dropped their old emotional baggage by the side of the road and simply walked away.

8. Heart Math

Heart Math is an app (computer, mobile phone, and tablet) that uses simple bio-feedback techniques, tools, and technologies to help minimize the effects of stress and anxiety. If you are familiar with smart phone and computer apps and you only have a few minutes each day to work on stress reduction, then Heart Math is a smart use of your time.

The HeartMath Inner Balance app and sensor work by replacing "the same old" negative responses to stress with feelings of confidence and ease. Heart-Math works by boosting the parasympathetic nervous system (the nervous system that calms the body) while decreasing the sympathetic nervous system (the system that gets you ready fight, run, or hide).

HeartMath improves focus, listening skills, and sleep — while decreasing anxiety, fatigue, and depression. Several studies have show that HeartMath enhances overall health, psychological health, and quality of life.

IMMUNE SYSTEM

	Problems	Solutions
IMMUNE SYSTEM	1. Immune diseases/disorders (your body attacks itself)	1. Consult a Functional Medicine doctor and test for depleted immune sys.
	2. Hidden Infections	2. Test & treat for infections
	3. Allergies	3. Test for food and environmental allergies
	4. Inflammation	4. Low-glycemic diet
	5. Hormone Imbalances	5. Test for hormone imbalances and treat them

Figure 4.6 outlines some major obstacles that prevent your immune system from healing your body from prostate diseases like BPH, prostatitis, and cancer.

Your immune system performs a complex balancing act between destroying invading organisms (bacteria, viruses, and other pathogens), perceived threats (foods, pollen, molds, yeasts, and so on), and preventing your defense systems from going haywire and attacking your own body, which can lead to auto-immune diseases.

An emergency room is an apt analogy for your immune system: Your immune system takes care of what it perceives to be biggest problems first. The more health issues you have, the fewer resources your immune system has to devote to each one.

If your immune system is already depleted because of multiple allergies, infections, and lots of chronic inflammation, then it doesn't have the reserves required to fight off a new problem (like prostate cancer).

If you have prostate cancer, at some point in your recent past, your immune system was too busy taking care of other ongoing (chronic) problems to rise to the occasion when your cancer was still in its infancy.

Here's the take-home message about your immune system: In order to heal from prostate disease (cancer), you have to start treating your body like a temple and taking care of your immune system so it can take care of you. Start by feeding your body what it needs (vegetables instead of sweet and starchy comfort foods), avoid any potential allergens (dietary or environmental), exercising daily, treat any chronic infections or diseases, start a daily stress reduction program, and have your hormones tested to see if your body is functioning well.

HORMONES

	Problems	Solutions
HORMONES	1. Unhealthy testosterone-to-estrogen ratio (not enough testosterone or too much estrogen)	1, 2. Test hormone levels & treat any imbalances
	2. Low levels of free or total testosterone	
	3. Immune system dysfunction	3. Find a good Functional Medicine doctor
	4. Metabolic issues	4. Get lean: Body fat produces estrogen
	5. Water stored in plastic bottles that leach estrogens	5, 6. Block environmental estrogens & avoid "estrogenic" foods
	6. Diet rich in soy and/or beer	
	7. Difficulty falling asleep or difficulty staying asleep	7. Find a good Functional Medicine doctor

Figure 4.7 gives a "tip of the iceberg" outline of how to maintain the healthy hormone levels and ratios that are essential to a healthy prostate. Ask your doctor about your male hormone levels and a program designed to optimize them.

Healthy hormone levels are essential for good prostate health and function. Hormones like testosterone, estrogen, DHT, and DHEA all play an interconnected role in the health of your prostate.

Contrary to outdated medical information that was once considered the bedrock truth about prostate cancer and prostate health, normal testosterone levels do NOT contribute to a man's risk of developing prostate cancer.

In fact, men with low testosterone levels (Low T) are at a greater his risk of developing prostate cancer. Recent medical studies continue to show that low testosterone:

- Does NOT protect men from prostate cancer
- INCREASES the risk of developing prostate cancer
- INCREASES the risk of developing the most aggressive kinds of prostate cancer (high-risk)

As with Low T, elevated estrogen levels (estrogen dominance) or a low testosterone-to-estrogen ratio can also increase your risk of developing prostate cancer.

The three simplest ways to lower your estrogen levels (and increase your testosterone-to-estrogen ratio) are to:

1. Get lean

2. Eliminate foods that contain estrogen and "estrogenic" (estrogen-like) compounds

3. Stop drinking water from plastic bottles.

Body fat produces a type of estrogen. If you reduce your amount of body fat, you will reduce your estrogen levels too. Cutting out soy products (soy milk, tofu, tempeh, soy protein, and miso) and hops (beer) will also shift your testosterone-to-estrogen ratio. Plastic bottles contain as many as 30 estrogen and estrogen-like compounds that leech into the water. Start drinking water from glass bottles instead.

We also recommend that you see a functional medical doctor and have your blood tested for these important hormones:

- Testosterone (free and total)
- DHT
- DHEA
- Estrogen

STRUCTURE

	Problems	Solutions
STRUCTURE	1. Sacral or lower back injuries and/or surgeries	1-6. Physical therapy, osteopathic manipulation, chiropractic, massage therapy, acupuncture, and MAT/NKT. (See **Page 109**)
	2. Loose ligaments in lower back and/or pelvis	
	3. Pelvic floor dysfunction	
	4. Pudendal nerve entrapment	1-6. Injection therapy such as PRP (Platelet Rich Plasma), stem cells, and Prolotherapy
	5. Poor posture	
	6. Organ and gland dysfunction within the bowl of the pelvis	

Figure 4.8 illustrates the impact of lower back and pelvic problems have on prostate disease and prostate cancer. If you have prostate issues and anatomical problems with your lower back or pelvis, please consider trying some of the "Hands-on Body Therapies" on **Page 109**.

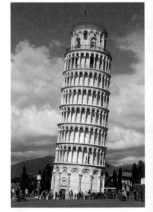

Your pelvic floor is an inter-woven web of muscles and connective tissues that form a "hammock" that keeps your intestines, urinary tract, and other internal organs in place. The best example we can think of to help you understand the importance of a healthy pelvic floor is the Leaning Tower of Pisa.

This famous leaning tower (where Galileo is said to have dropped two cannonballs to study the effect of mass on the speed of falling objects) doesn't lean because the tower is tilted. *It leans because the foundation is sinking on one side of the tower more than it is on the other.*

Think of your pelvic floor like the foundation beneath the Tower of Pisa. If the foundation of your pelvis is, injured, tilted, too tight, too loose, or too tight in some areas and loose in others, then (like the part of the tower that is above ground) the organs inside your pelvis are at a greater risk of all sorts of structural complications.

Although pelvic floor problems are largely responsible for these complications, the real culprit usually lies in the structural integrity of the lower back and ligaments that

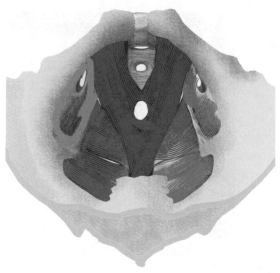

Figure 4.9 Illustrates a bird's-eye view of a healthy pelvic floor — a web of interconnected tissue that supports all the organs and glands of pelvis and lower abdomen — including the prostate.

connect the pelvis to the spine (iliolumbar ligaments) and hold the pelvis together (sacroiliac ligaments).

Spinal injuries, herniated discs, broken vertebrae or pelvic bones, spinal stenosis (diminished disc space), spinal surgeries, scoliosis, and other conditions can also interfere with the nerves that go to the pelvic floor and organs inside the "bowl" of your pelvis. (See **Figure 4.9**)

Pelvic floor problems can affect everything from circulation, muscular strength, urinary function, digestion, inflammation, infections ... to your ability to have and maintain an erection. In other words, the health of your lower back, pelvis, and pelvic floor have a huge impact on health of your prostate.

Unlike changing your diet, getting more exercise, or learning to meditate — resolving pelvic floor, lower back, and other pelvic issues requires help from a skilled professional trained in hands-on body therapies such as:

- Physical Therapy
- Chiropractic manipulation
- Osteopathic medicine
- Acupuncture
- Rolfing
- Touch for Health
- Muscle Activation Technique (MAT)
- Neurokinetic Therapy (NKT)

TOXIC SUBSTANCES

	Problems	Solutions
TOXIC SUBSTANCES	1. From sources outside your body: soap, shampoo, cleansers, disinfectants, harsh chemicals, pesticides, herbicides, fungicides, fertilizers, heavy metals, and chemicals used in warfare like Agent Orange.	1. Remove all harsh chemicals from your home: cleansers, pesticides, herbicides, fungicides, and so on.
	2. Manufactured inside your body: Toxic substances usually created by bacteria and other microbes that live inside your body.	1, 2. Eat organic fruits and vegetables — or at least non-GMO food.
	3. Cannot be excreted: Toxins/toxic substances that your body is unable to excrete through normal channels: liver, intestines, lungs, kidneys, and skin.	1, 3. Work with a Functional Medicine Doctor to improve your body's ability to get rid of toxins through normal pathways of excretion.
	4. Poorly functioning immune system and long-term allergies.	1, 4 & 5. Seek professional medical help from the best specialists you can afford.
	5. Organ problems: liver, kidneys, lungs, heart, intestines, or skin.	

Figure 4.10 outlines how toxic substances come in three categories based on their origin and whether your body can process them: 1. From outside your body, 2. Made within your body, 3. Cannot be excreted by your body.

"Toxins" is a word that gets tossed around a lot by people who use "cleanses and fasts" as a form of self-purification. In that context, "toxins" may mean anything from the chemicals in household cleansers to weed killers to the byproducts of having a second helping of dessert and drinking too much wine last weekend.

Please don't misunderstand us: there are hundreds of peer-reviewed scientific papers that support the medicinal benefits of cleanses and fasts — especially intermittent fasting (micro-fasts) that last 12-16 hours.

For the purposes of this discussion, however, we will use the term "toxic substances" to mean both biological "toxins" (biochemicals produced by plants, animals or microbes that include spider bites, poison ivy, and the bacteria that causes botulism) and "environmental toxins" (industrial chemicals and heavy metals), as well as synthetic chemicals (pesticides, herbicides, and fungicides).

To these two groups, we should also add the ingredients of certain pharmaceutical medications. These are the ingredients that cause the problems mentioned at the end of TV commercials: "In some cases, people who take XYZ may experience..."

Essentially, we are talking about chemicals that your body is poorly equipped to metabolize or excrete. These chemicals come from three sources:

1. Outside your body
   (environmental toxins/toxic substances)
2. Biochemical
   (substances manufactured within your body)
3. Chemicals that cannot be excreted (usually toxins/ toxic substances that came from outside your body)

Because your body (mostly your lungs, liver, kidneys, intestines, and skin) has a hard time getting rid of toxic chemicals, these substances become trapped in your tissues, wreaking havoc on the microscopic, cellular, organ, and whole-body levels.

As your organs work overtime to get rid of these chemicals, the extra load weakens the organs (and the immune system) and prevents them from performing their normal functions of cleansing and detoxifying your body.

So what can you do (short of moving to a deserted island) to eliminate your exposure to these toxic substances?

Here are a few simple ideas:

- Purchase organic and non-GMO food
- Dispose of all household cleaners and other products that contain ingredients you cannot pronounce, and replace them with natural soap, baking soda, vinegar, and citrus solvents.
- Dispose of all herbicides, pesticides, and fungicides in your garage, basement, attic, or under the kitchen sink.
- Purchase bottled water in glass bottles or install a home water filtration system.

THE PROSTATE CANCER PERFECT STORM

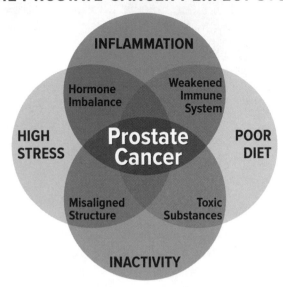

Figure 4.11 displays the "Perfect Storm" of the seven health factors that create inflammation and increase the risk of prostate cancer. Obviously, factors like age, family history, other illnesses, and ethnicity also play a role in this diagram.

INFLAMMATION MANAGEMENT SUMMARY

Getting rid of inflammation is a complex subject that requires more information than we can possibly present in a single chapter of this book. Here is a quick list of the top eight action steps we recommend (one for each health factor listed in this chapter — plus inflammation).

1. Inflammation: Treat prostatitis, BPH, and PIN.

2. Diet: Read food labels and reduce your consumption of all sweeteners, trans fats, and processed foods.

3. Inactivity: Walk, run, ride a bike, swim, hike, go to the gym, but raise your heart rate for 30 minutes every day.

4. Stress: Spend 20 minutes a day practicing stress reduction: prayer, meditation, Chi Gong, or Heart Math.

5. Immune System: Get treatment for all chronic allergies, lingering infections, and autoimmune disorders.

6. Hormones: Avoid all estrogens, estrogenic foods & beverages (soy & hops), and pseudo-estrogens in food storage containers (plastic bags and bottles).

7. Structure: Get evaluated for "pelvic floor dysfunction" by a physical therapist or other knowledgeable therapist.

8. Toxic Substances: Eat organic food & drink finely filtered water (not just water from a charcoal filter).

Doctor Story
DR. PHRANQ TAMBURRI, NMD

Naturopathic Medicine

Longevity Medical

Phoenix, Arizona

I'm not in the business of telling people what to do. I am in the business of asking questions, listening, evaluating answers, and making suggestions based on those answers.

I built my practice around four questions:

1. What's the chance of you having clinically significant prostate cancer that is confined inside the gland and will be found at the same location in multiple prostate biopsies?

To answer that question, we usually have a long conversation about how we all have cancer in our bodies, Gleason scores, the number of prostate cancer cells replicating, the spectrum of PSA tests, Doppler MRI, digital rectal exams, which leads to the money question...

2. What's the chance that your prostate cancer will kill you in the next 5 years?

If your cancer is not metastatic, at what point will it cross the line and escape your prostate: 10 years, 20 years ... longer? In other words, what is your cancer's "metabolic momentum"? Predicting metabolic momentum is an amalgam of Gleason score, family & medical history, biopsy, PSA, and several other tests.

3. What else is adding to your PSA?

We need to know what we're treating. Besides prostate cancer, the #1 reason for a high PSA is prostatitis; the #2 reason is BPH. Most men have two or more going on at the same time.

4. How do we track your cancer over time?

Prostate cancer is like a polar bear: It can be a ferocious papa bear or a cute little cub. If we are trying to treat the bear and it's on an iceberg (BPH) in the middle of a blizzard (prostatitis), we've got to get the bear on land and stop the storm before we can treat it. If a patient has all three going on and his PSA falls, which one of the three improved?

LOOKING AHEAD

CHAPTER 1: You or your doctor is concerned about your prostate — We provide you with **Prostate 101**: where it lives, what it does, plus relevant statistics.

CHAPTER 2: Your doctor told you to **schedule a prostate biopsy** — We give you a **Prostate Biopsy Assessment Tool** to see if you actually need one, and what to expect if you do.

CHAPTER 3: You have a prostate biopsy — We explain the steps you need to take, whether you have a **negative biopsy or a positive biopsy**.

CHAPTER 4: You want to **use your cancer diagnosis as a springboard to better health** — We help you address your wellness goals with a proven plan that covers inflammation, diet, exercise, stress, immune system, hormone optimization, anatomy, and removing toxic substances.

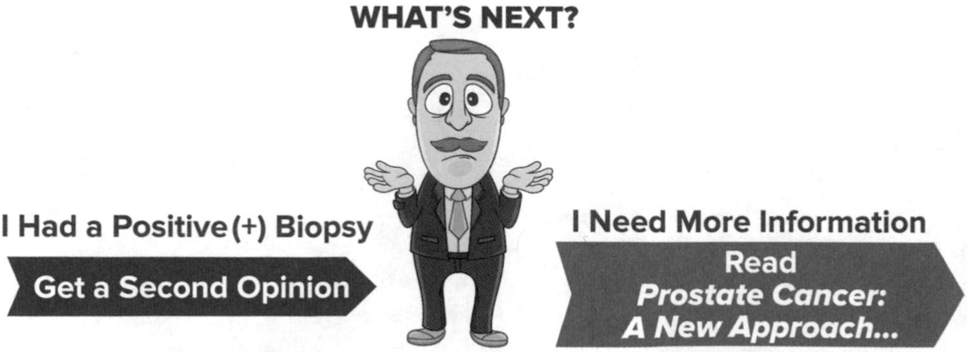

WHAT'S NEXT?

I Had a Positive (+) Biopsy

Get a Second Opinion

I Need More Information

Read
***Prostate Cancer:
A New Approach...***

WELCOME TO THE TOOLBOX
CHAPTER 4 **TOOLBOX**

THE **CHAPTER 4** TOOLBOX ALLOWS YOU TO APPLY THE SEVEN HEALTH FACTORS THAT DECREASE INFLAMMATION AND REDUCE THE RISK OF PROSTATE CANCER. THE GOAL HERE IS TO HELP YOU REGAIN YOUR OVERALL HEALTH AND THE HEALTH OF YOUR PROSTATE:

1. **Diet**
2. **Inactivity**
3. **Stress**
4. **Immune System**
5. **Hormones**
6. **Structure**
7. **Toxic Substances**

The **Chapter 4 Toolbox** gives you the opportunity to put the information presented in this chapter to work for you right away.

The beauty of the seven health areas listed above (plus inflammation) is that they will benefit anyone; however, they are designed for men who have been recently diagnosed with prostate disease, especially cancer.

Regardless of your diagnosis, the kind of cancer you have, your age, or the type of treatment you select, you can make changes in these seven health areas immediately and begin to receive their benefits.

Will they cure cancer? That depends upon which kind of cancer you have, how much, where, and a host of other factors.

If you look at **Figure 4.12** starting on **Page 117**, you'll see two empty spaces at the end of each section that say: "pick two causes listed above" and "pick two treatments listed above."

These spaces allow you to choose two of the bullet points listed in each health area and begin working on them. Some of the actions are simple: Walk away from your desk every 20 minutes and take a lap around the office. (You can set your watch or phone to remind you.) Other actions are more complicated: Change your diet, start exercising, or have your hormones levels tested.

As with all things in this book, begin at a pace that works for you. If shifting your diet and exercise habits is all you can handle, start there.

On **Page 112** we also included our top 8 actions steps we recommend for each health area.

Remember: It's more important to get started and stay on your path than it is to procrastinate about picking the perfect actions. So, let's get started.

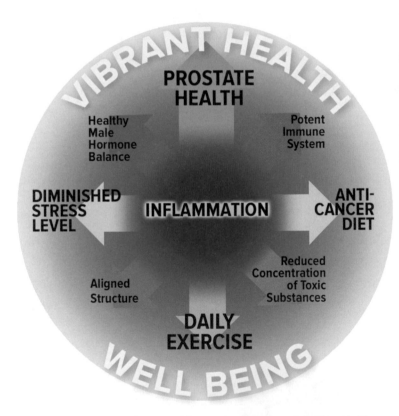

Figure 4.2 reverses the elements of the seven point plan we introduced in **Figure 4.0** at the beginning of the chapter. As you can see, if you reverse the direction of the seven health factors (plus inflammation) so they move towards health and well being, you reverse the course of your condition.

	CAUSES	SOLUTIONS
INFLAMMATION	1. Immune System	1. Treat infections & prostatitis
	2. Diet	2. Eat a low-glycemic (low-sugar) diet
	3. Toxic Substances	3. See **Page 110**
	4. Inactivity	4. Exercise 30 minutes a day
	5. Structure	5. See **Page 108**
	6. Stress	6. Start a stress reduction program
	7. Hormones	7. Have your hormone levels and ratios checked by a certified functional medicine doctor
	8. Prostate	8. Begin our 7-point program
	PICK TWO CAUSES LISTED ABOVE.	**PICK TWO SOLUTIONS LISTED ABOVE.**
DIET	1. Insulin/sugar problems & toxic chemicals in food	1. Eat mostly organic vegetables (especially cruciferous vegetables) and fruit
	2. High-glycemic diet	2. Low-glycemic diet
	3. Growth hormone/antibiotics in food	3. Eat animal protein that is free of all hormones and antibiotics
	4. Processed foods and trans fats	4. Restore the balance between omega 3 & omega 6 fatty acids
	5. Grains	5. Limit grains and breads
	6. Poor quality oils	6. Use more olive and coconut oil
	7. Alcohol, sweetened sodas, and caffeine consumption	7. Limit alcohol, sodas, and caffeine
	PICK TWO CAUSES LISTED ABOVE.	**PICK TWO SOLUTIONS LISTED ABOVE.**

Figure 4.12 (above and on the following pages) gives you the opportunity to use the seven health factors from **Chapter 4** (plus inflammation) and select four aspects from each heading that you would like to use as a springboard to improve your health. We invite you to use the space below each heading to write down two causes of dis-ease that you want to change, as well as two solutions you are willing to implement.

TOOLBOX

TOOLBOX

	CAUSES	SOLUTIONS
INACTIVITY	1. Chronic inflammation, pain, and habitual stress	1-3. Move your body: Stand up every hour, walk around, do chores, stay active
	2. Accumulation of toxic substances in excess body fat leads to being both overweight and unhealthy	1-3. Build your strength, endurance, and flexibility slowly over time. Exercise daily but avoid overtraining.
	3. Lack of exercise leads to stagnant circulation, fatigue, depression, and a diminished desire to move your body	1-3. Combine slow/steady exercise with resistance training and interval training, which improves circulation and removal of toxic substances
	PICK TWO CAUSES LISTED ABOVE.	**PICK TWO SOLUTIONS LISTED ABOVE.**
STRESS	1. A prostate cancer diagnosis	1. The "right fit" prostate cancer treatment plan
	2. Fears about money and your close relationships	2. Seek sound financial support and open up to the people closest to you
	3. Work-related issues	3. Talk with co-workers and supervisors (if you can)
	4. Feeling overwhelmed	4. Daily deep breathing practice promotes feeling calm
	5. Too much cortisol and adrenaline in your system	5. Daily exercise, limit stimulants, prayer/meditation
	PICK TWO CAUSES LISTED ABOVE.	**PICK TWO SOLUTIONS LISTED ABOVE.**
IMMUNE SYSTEM	1. Immune diseases/disorder (your body attacks itself)	1. Consult a Functional Medicine doctor and test for depleted immune system
	2. Hidden Infections	2. Test & treat for infections
	3. Allergies	3. Test for food and environmental allergies
	4. Inflammation	4. Low-glycemic diet
	5. Hormone Imbalances	5. Test for hormone imbalances and treat them
	PICK TWO CAUSES LISTED ABOVE.	**PICK TWO SOLUTIONS LISTED ABOVE.**

	CAUSES	SOLUTIONS
HORMONES	1. Unhealthy testosterone-to-estrogen ratio (not enough testosterone or too much estrogen)	1, 2. Test hormone levels & treat any imbalances
	2. Low levels of free or total testosterone	
	3. Immune system dysfunction	3. Find a good Functional Medicine doctor
	4. Metabolic issues	4. Get lean: Body fat produces estrogen
	5. Water stored in plastic bottles that leach estrogens	5, 6. Block environmental estrogens & avoid "estrogenic" foods
	6. Diet rich in soy and/or beer	
	7. Difficulty falling asleep or difficulty staying asleep	7. Find a good Functional Medicine doctor
	PICK TWO CAUSES LISTED ABOVE.	**PICK TWO SOLUTIONS LISTED ABOVE.**
STRUCTURE	1. Sacral or low back injuries and/or surgeries	1-6. Physical therapy, osteopathic manipulation, chiropractic, massage therapy, acupuncture, and MAT/NKT
	2. Loose ligaments in lower back and/or pelvis	
	3. Pelvic floor dysfunction	1-6. Injection therapy such as PRP (Platelet Rich Plasma), stem cells, and Prolotherapy
	4. Pudendal nerve entrapment	
	5. Poor posture	
	6. Organ and gland dysfunction within the bowl of the pelvis	
	PICK TWO CAUSES LISTED ABOVE.	**PICK TWO SOLUTIONS LISTED ABOVE.**

	CAUSES	SOLUTIONS
TOXIC SUBSTANCES	1. From sources outside your body: cleansers, disinfectants, harsh chemicals, pesticides, herbicides, fungicides, fertilizers, heavy metals, and chemicals used in warfare like Agent Orange	1. Remove all harsh chemicals from your home: pesticides, herbicides, fungicides, and so on. 1. Replace household cleaners with simple solutions like vinegar, baking soda, citrus solvents, and soap.
	2. Manufactured inside your body: Toxic substances usually manufactured by bacteria and other microbes that live inside your body	1, 2. Eat organic fruits and vegetables — or at least non-GMO food.
	3. Cannot be excreted: Toxins/toxic substances that your body is unable to excrete through normal channels: liver, intestines, lungs, kidneys, and skin.	1, 3. Work with a Functional Medicine Doctor to improve your body's ability to get rid of toxins through normal pathways of excretion.
	4. Poorly functioning immune system and long-term allergies.	1, 4 & 5. Seek professional medical help from the best specialists you can afford to see.
	5. Organ problems: liver, kidneys, lungs, heart, intestines, or skin.	
	PICK TWO CAUSES LISTED ABOVE.	**PICK TWO SOLUTIONS LISTED ABOVE.**

WHAT IS FUNCTIONAL MEDICINE?

According to the Institute for Functional Medicine, "Functional Medicine addresses the underlying causes of disease, using a systems-oriented approach and engaging both patient and practitioner in a therapeutic partnership. It is an evolution in the practice of medicine that better addresses the healthcare needs of the 21st century."

HOW IS FUNCTIONAL MEDICINE DIFFERENT?

Functional Medicine integrates the latest scientific information with lifestyle and environmental factors to create a new medical system that allows healthcare professionals to better understand what each patient needs.

WHERE TO FIND A FUNCTIONAL MEDICAL DOCTOR IN YOUR AREA

For more information about Functional Medicine and Functional Medical doctors in your area, we invite you to visit the following websites:

http://www.abihm.org
http://www.abihm.org/search-doctors
https://www.functionalmedicine.org

TOOLBOX

GUIDE TO EATING OUT

Restaurants

1. Say, "No thank you" to the bread or chips and salsa that automatically arrive on your table. These high-glycemic carbs are metabolized just like sugar. You are essentially "packing on the pounds" before your meal arrives.
2. Start your meal with a small salad. Salads usually arrive first and take the edge off your hunger, and your meal has a healthy start.
3. Consider ordering several side dishes or something from the "a la Carte" menu. That way, you can *get your vegetables* and still feel satisfied.
4. Avoid "all you can eat" buffet-style restaurants. They promote overeating.
5. Skip dessert. You will feel lighter, look thinner, and have fewer health issues.

Parties

1. Eat a healthy mini-meal before you go. Include some veggies, protein, and healthy fats. Try a simple spring-mix salad with some chicken or canned tuna, sprinkle in a few seeds or nuts, and add half an avocado. It takes under 10 minutes to prepare.
2. Bring a couple of bottles of sparkling water.
3. Alcoholic beverages are the kings of "empty calories." Alcohol is metabolized into fat in your liver, and alcohol is a carcinogen. Best to avoid it. If you drink alcohol, alternate between alcoholic beverages and sparkling water.
4. Arrive a little late. You'll spend less time "grazing" the finger food.
5. Bring a healthy side dish or appetizer. That way, you have a go-to item — instead of nachos, pizza, Buffalo chicken wings, or seven-layer dip.

At Work

1. Bring your own lunch. This practice will you save $5-10/day, and give you more control over what you eat. You also won't find yourself staring at a vending machine at 3:30, trying to decide between a Snickers bar or bag of Cheetos.
2. Eat less bread. You'll lose weight and lower your insulin production. Make yourself an open-faced sandwich. If you eat out, order a lettuce or tortilla wrap.
3. Avoid sweetened energy drinks. If you feel run down, have an unsweetened cup of coffee or tea. If your job allows, go for a 10-minute walk instead.
4. Bring your own bottled water (unless your work provides it). Think Flint, Mich. Avoid the estrogen by drinking water from glass bottles whenever possible.
5. Avoid crashing and burning by keeping a ready supply of healthy snacks in your desk, locker, or car: nuts, seeds, low-glycemic fruit, and bottled water.

TOOLBOX

NOTES:

TOOLBOX

GLOSSARY

4Kscore Test - The 4Kscore Test is a blood test that ranks a man's risk for having aggressive prostate cancer.

AUA Score - A questionnaire that helps men quantify their urinary symptoms and their treatment(s). Also known as the International Prostate Symptom Score (IPSS).

Benign Prostatic Hyperplasia (BPH) - BPH is an enlarged prostate gland. If an enlarged prostate pinches off the urethra, it can cause urinary problems.

Bio-individuality - The concept that each person's biochemical make-up is unique (non-identical), even with identical twins. This includes biochemical process from nutritional requirements to the proteins that DNA instructs individual cells to make.

Bladder - A mucular organ that stores the urine produced by the kidneys before it is excreted.

Bone Scan - A type of X-ray that is used to determine if prostate cancer has spread to the bones.

Brainspotting - A somatic therapy for reducing anxiety, fear, and Post Traumatic Stress Disorder (PTSD)

CAT Scan (Computerized Axial Tomography Scan) - A painless form of X-rays that generates cross-sectional views of a patient's body.

ConfirmMDx - a biopsy based test that helps doctors rule out the need for a repeat biopsy or indicate the presence of "hidden cancer" that a previous biopsy missed.

Cortisol - A steroid hormone produced by the adrenal gland in response to stress or low blood sugar. Cortisol is also called "hydrocortisone" when used as a medication.

DHEA - An adrenal gland hormone that is a precursor of both male and female sex hormones.

DHT - This powerful male sex hormone is the most important male hormone inside the prostate, where DHT has a 5-10 times greater affinity for male sex hormone receptors than testosterone.

Digital Rectal Exam (DRE) - A procedure where a doctor inserts a gloved finger (digit) into the rectum in order to examine the prostate through the thin muscular wall of the rectum.

DNA (deoxyribonucleic acid) - The building blocks of life on Earth. Long strands of DNA, called "genes," determine everything from skin color to the likelihood of developing prostate cancer.

EMDR - Eye Movement Desensitization and Reprocessing is a psychotherapy technique for treating disturbing memories and PTSD.

Emotional Freedom Technique (Tapping) - A form of somatic therapy that integrates acupuncture, neuro-linguistic programming, and other treatments to release negative emotions and unwanted habits.

Epigenetic Testing - Tests that use tissue samples from a prostate biopsy look for biomarkers that indicate the presence (or absence) of prostate cancer.

Erectile Dysfunction (ED) - The inability to have or maintain an erection.

Extracapsular Extension - Prostate cancer that extends into or beyond the capsule (membrane) of the prostate.

GLOSSARY CONTINUED

False Negative - A negative result for a test, like a prostate biopsy, that failed to detect the presence cancer.

Genetic Testing - Tests that look for certain genetic markers in cancer cells taken from tissue samples, like a prostate biopsy. These markers indicate how aggressive the cancer is.

Gene - A portion of a DNA molecule that controls the development of one or more physical traits (heredity) or physiological responses (the likelihood of developing one or more traits).

Gleason Score - A method that pathologists use to determine how aggressive a certain sample of prostate cancer is. A Gleason score includes two numbers, which are added together to produce a sum. For example, 3 + 4 = 7.

GMO: Genetically Modified Organism - Any living organism, typically crops and vegetables, that are modified for enhanced to modify certain traits, like crop yield.

Hormones - A substance created by a gland, which circulates in the blood and stimulates the cells of different organs, glands, or tissues.

Imaging- X-rays, MRI, CAT scans, ultrasound, and other similar diagnostic tests.

Insulin - The hormone that moves sugar from the blood into the cells of the body where it can be metabolized as fuel or stored for future use.

Lab Tests - Blood, urine, and tissue sample tests used to determine the presence (or absence) of prostate cancer.

Lumbosacral - The lowest part of the back where the end of the lumbar spine meets the sacrum.

Lymph Node - A network of small pockets along the lymphatic system where lymph (also called "plasma" or "serum") is filtered and lymphocytes (white blood cells) are made.

Magnetic Resonance Imaging (MRI) - a type of imaging that uses magnetic fields and radio waves to create detailed images of the organs and tissues.

Methylation - A higher than normal concentration of methyl groups (CH_3) in a tissue sample, which indicates the presence of prostate cancer.

MRI Fusion Prostate Biopsy - A type of prostate biopsy that overlays an MRI image of the prostate on top of a standard ultrasound image, allowing for pinpoint accuracy and the ability to sample the same spot in the prostate multiple times.

Mutation - Any alteration in DNA structure or sequence that may be transmitted to future generations.

Needle Cores - The tissue samples collected during a prostate biopsy.

Neuromodulation Technique - The alteration of nerve activity through the delivery of electrical stimulation or chemical agents to targeted sites of the body.

PCA3 - A urine test for a particular gene that is only found in prostate cancer cells. The PCA3 test is not affected by prostate size (BPH), PSA, or prostatitis.

Pelvic Floor - An interwoven web of muscles and connective tissues that form a hammock that supports the intestines, urinary tract, and other internal organs.

PIN - a pre-cancerous condition that causes the prostate's epithelial cells (cells that line the small sacs inside the prostate) to undergo microscopic changes.

GLOSSARY CONTINUED

PNI - Cancer that has spread into the space that surrounds a nerve.

Prostate Biopsy - An in-office procedure that looks for prostate cancer by taking 12-24 small tissue samples, which are then analyzed under a microscope.

Prostate Cancer - A disease of the prostate gland in which cells develop abnormally. These abnormal cells can form tumors, grow at an uncontrollable rate, and spread throughout the body.

Prostate Zones - The prostate is divided into 3 zones: Central, Peripheral, and Transitional.

Prostatitis - An inflammation of the prostate.

PSA (Prostate Specific Antigen) - A protein produced by the prostate that helps transport and nourish sperm after ejaculation. A certain amount of PSA leaks into the blood stream and is detectable by a PSA blood test.

PSA Density - A measurement of PSA that factors in the size of a man's prostate. (Bigger prostates leak more PSA into the blood stream.)

PSA Free - PSA that is NOT attached (bound) to any proteins. A higher concentration of Free PSA indicates a lower likelihood of prostate cancer.

PSA Testing - A blood test that detects the concentration of PSA.

PSA Total - A measurement of PSA Free + PSA bound to other proteins.

PSA Velocity - The rate of rise (or fall) of any PSA number over time.

Rectum - The final straight portion of the intestines that ends at the anus.

Sacroiliac - The two hinge joints that occur between the major bones of the pelvis: the sacrum and the ilium.

Seminal Vesicle - A pair of two small glands that connect to the top of the prostate and produce about 70 percent of the fluid in semen (seminal fluid).

Seminal Vesicle Fluid - The fluid produced by the seminal vesicles during ejaculation.

Seminal Vesicle Involvement - Prostate cancer that has spread to the seminal vesicles.

Standard American Diet - A style of eating characterized by a high intake of sugar, processed foods, red meat, processed meat, high-fat dairy products, refined grains, simple carbohydrates — and an absence of fresh fruits and vegetables.

TRUS (standard) Biopsy - A standard ultrasound-guided prostate biopsy. Also called a "Random" biopsy because of this procedure's lack of accuracy.

TURP - A type of surgery (rotor-rooter) to relieve the urinary symptoms caused by "BPH" (see above).

Ultrasound - The most common type of imaging used during a prostate biopsy.

Urethra - The tube by which urine flows from the bladder to the end of the penis.

Urinary Frequency - The feeling of having to urinate frequently.

Urinary Retention - Being unable to completely empty the bladder.

Urinary Sphincter - Another name for the "Pelvic Floor" (see above).

Urinary Stricture - Scar tissue that forms in the urethra.

Urinary Urgency - The feeling of having to urinate "right now"!

Western Diet - See "Standard American Diet"

INDEX

ABOUT THE AUTHORS

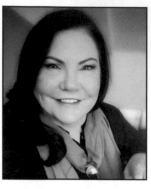

EMILIA RIPOLL, MD - Dr. Ripoll has been practicing urology and urologic oncology in the Denver metro area for more than 25 years.

Born in Barcelona, Spain and educated in the United States, Dr. Ripoll graduated from the University of Colorado School of Medicine with honors, did her residency and post-doctorate fellowship at Baylor College of Medicine, and received her medical acupuncture training at UCLA.

As an American Urological Association Foundation Scholar, Dr. Ripoll researched genetic predisposition and the role of proto-oncogenes in the development of prostate cancer.

For more information about Emilia Ripoll, visit emiliaripollmd.com

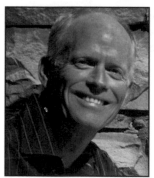

MARK SAUNDERS is a writer, editor, and 10-year cancer survivor. As an active surveillance prostate cancer patient, Mark did not receive traditional treatment like surgery or some form of radiation. Instead, he dramatically overhauled his lifestyle — and his cancer went away — and hasn't come back since.

As a prostate cancer survivor, Mark has dedicated his life to sharing what he has learned about health and wellness. A journey that he calls, "Inside out, round-about, and back again."

For more information about Mark Saunders, visit markbsaunders.com

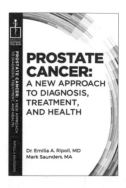

Dr. Emilia Ripoll and Mark Saunders are also the authors of *Prostate Cancer: A New Apporach to Diagnosis, Treatment, and Health* — a greatly expanded version of *Do You Have Prostate Cancer?* for men who have received a prostate cancer diagnosis. This book includes six additional chapters and two special sections. Visit health-otb.com for more information.

NOTES:

NOTES: